Practice Workbook of
MEDICAL SURGICAL NURSING

Practice Workbook of
MEDICAL SURGICAL NURSING

BT Basavanthappa MN PhD

Principal
RajaRajeswari College of Nursing
Bengaluru, Karnataka, India

Former Professor and Principal
Government College of Nursing
Bengaluru, Karnataka, India

PhD Guide for Research Work
Ex-Member
Faculty of Nursing, RGUHS, Karnataka, India
Academic Council, RGUHS, Karnataka, India
Examiner
UG, PG and Doctoral Degree Courses on Nursing in various Universities
Ex-Program In-Charge
IGNOU, BSc (N) Course, Karnataka and Goa, India
Life Member
Nursing Research Society of India, New Delhi, India
Trained Nurses Association of India, New Delhi, India
President
RGUHS, Nursing Teachers Association, Karnataka, India
Winner
Bharat Excellence Award and Gold Medal
Vikas Rattan Gold Award
UWA Lifetime Achievement Award
Shree Veeranjaneya 'Shrujanashri' Award

JAYPEE The Health Sciences Publisher
New Delhi | London | Philadelphia | Panama

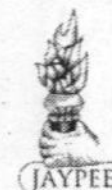

Jaypee Brothers Medical Publishers (P) Ltd

Headquarters

Jaypee Brothers Medical Publishers (P) Ltd
4838/24, Ansari Road, Daryaganj
New Delhi 110 002, India
Phone: +91-11-43574357
Fax: +91-11-43574314
Email: jaypee@jaypeebrothers.com

Overseas Offices

J.P. Medical Ltd
83 Victoria Street, London
SW1H 0HW (UK)
Phone: +44 20 3170 8910
Fax: +44 (0) 20 3008 6180
Email: info@jpmedpub.com

Jaypee-Highlights Medical Publishers Inc
City of Knowledge, Bld. 237, Clayton
Panama City, Panama
Phone: +1 507-301-0496
Fax: +1 507-301-0499
Email: cservice@jphmedical.com

Jaypee Medical Inc
The Bourse
111 South Independence Mall East
Suite 835, Philadelphia, PA 19106, USA
Phone: +1 267-519-9789
Email: jpmed.us@gmail.com

Jaypee Brothers Medical Publishers (P) Ltd
17/1-B Babar Road, Block-B, Shaymali
Mohammadpur, Dhaka-1207
Bangladesh
Mobile: +08801912003485
Email: jaypeedhaka@gmail.com

Jaypee Brothers Medical Publishers (P) Ltd
Bhotahity, Kathmandu
Nepal
Phone: +977-9741283608
Email: kathmandu@jaypeebrothers.com

Website: www.jaypeebrothers.com
Website: www.jaypeedigital.com

Inquiries for bulk sales may be solicited at: jaypee@jaypeebrothers.com

Practice Workbook of Medical Surgical Nursing

First Edition: **2015**

ISBN 978-93-5152-588-2

Printed at Sanat Printers, Kundli

Preface

It gives me immense pleasure and satisfaction to introduce the *Practice Workbook of Medical Surgical Nursing,* which will enable the students to meet their practical requirements of the concerned subject.

Nursing is an applied science, but the knowledge related to the subject has been taught in the classroom. The application of the knowledge of nursing is essential for all nursing students, for which, there is a need for every student to undergo a real practical experience in hospitals or healthcare institutions. The main objective of clinical experience is that the students will be able to understand, comprehend, correlate theory with practice and develop various skills in performing various activities related to nursing.

My aim of designing this book is to acquaint all nursing students with knowledge and skill in providing proper nursing care to clients, who come in their practical settings.

This 'Practice Workbook' can be used as clinical record of experience in the area of medical surgical nursing, which will help the students to write their prescribed assignments.

I have tried my best to provide basic instructions and guidelines to prepare their assignments in a proper way.

I hope this book will be beneficial to the students in their selected nursing courses.

BT Basavanthappa

Contents

PHOTOGRAPH

STUDENTS PROFILE

Name of the College : ....

....

Name of the Student : ....

Registration No : ....

Age and Date of Birth : .... Religion: ....

Father's Name : ....

Mother's Name : ....

Mother Tongue : .... Batch: ....

Date of Joining the Course : ....

Date of Starting of Clinical Posting : ....

Date of Completion of Clinical Posting : ....

Permanent Address : ....

....

Signature of the Student **Signature of the HOD**

Signature of the Principal

Signature of the Internal Examiner **Signature of the External Examiner**

INSTRUCTIONS TO STUDENTS

1. Students must wear the uniform, shoes and socks prescribed by the Institution/College.
2. Students must have prescribed pocket articles required during clinical experience, i.e. small scissors, color pens, pocket note book, rulers, etc.
3. Students are required to groomed their hairs and nails properly.
4. Students are not expected to wear jewelries except wrist watch with second hand.
5. Students are expected to wear gowns, bonnets, masks and caps, in the area of hospital where it is needed as per the policy of the hospital.
6. Students are not expected to use telephones, cellular/mobile phones, pocket radios and other electronic media during clinical hours, while on duty.
7. Students are not expected to allow any of their visitors during clinical hours in the premises of setting, i.e. hospital, healthcare institution.
8. Students are prohibited from entering vacant rooms/unoccupied rooms of the hospital unless it is official or justifiable.
9. Students are expected to be in the ward/unit/special unit. Remain in respective areas during the prescribed hours and not to roaming around other wards/units unnecessarily.
10. Students are expected to leave the ward by informing Clinical Supervisor or Staff Nurse during emergencies.
11. Students are expected to take care of their individual client/patient properly by applying nursing process promptly.
12. Students are expected to maintain punctuality, sincerity in attending clinical experience in the hospital or any healthcare institution.
13. Students are expected to maintain honesty, punctuality, sincerity, in dealing with the patients.
14. Students are expected to maintain promptness and show interest in learning various skills during the posting of clinical experiences and learn the skills properly.
15. Student who shows misbehavior like dishonesty, uncourtesy, forgery, immoral conduct, loitering, using dangerous drugs, alcohol, smoking and others not tolerated, if so they will be punished accordingly to policies of the Government or Management of the Institution.
16. Students are instructed that when preparing or performing any procedure on patient, prior permission from Supervisor/Ward in Charge/Staff Nurse is needed.
17. Students are instructed complete their assignments and procedures of clinical experience during clinical posting in stipulated time and get signature from respective teachers.
18. Students are instructed to read the Guidelines for Reporting, History Taking, Physical Examination, Application of Nursing of Process, Nursing Care Plan and Others.

SECTION I

CASE 1

HISTORY TAKING

(ē Guidelines to Report History Taking)

BIOGRAPHICAL DATA

Name of the Patient: ....

Name of the Father/Guardian/Husband: ....

Age: .... Date of Birth: .... Sex: ....

Marital Status: .... Education: .... Occupation: ....

Monthly Income: ....

Mother Tongue: .... Religion: .... Nationality: ....

Educational Status: ....

Date of Admission: .... IP No: .... MLC/OP No: ....

Address: ....

....

....

Medical Diagnosis: .... Doctor's Name: ....

Name of the Hospital: ....

Ward: .... Bed Number: ....

Date of Data Collection: ....

Present History of Illness (Medical Surgical)

Give brief notes of onset of symptoms, their frequency, exact location of distress, character of complaints, e.g. intensity of pain, quality of sputum, emesis or discharge, etc.

For example: ....

....

....

....

....

....

....

Past History of Illness (Medical Surgical)

Mention brief note of history of childhood illnesses, childhood immunization, allergies, accidental injuries, hospitalization of serious illness, treatment given, complications and medication prescribed if anything that are in relevant to present health and disease.

....

....

....

Personal History

1. **Habits:** Substance use and abuse (i.e. tobacco, alcohol, coffee, tea, illicit or recreational drug, etc.) such as smoking, tobacco chewing, drug addiction (if present daily/occasionally, duration of use, exercises and yoga, etc.

   For example: Smoking: Yes/No: .... Per day: .... No. of years: ....
   Tobacco chewing: ....
   Alcohol: .... Drug addict (specify): ....
   ....
   ....

2. **Diet:** Members about typical diet, vegetarian and non-vegetarian/pattern of taking of meals:
   - Vegetarian: .... No of meals per day: ....
   - Any allergic to any food items: ....
3. **Sleep and rest pattern:**
   - Timing of sleep: .... Duration: ....
   - Timing of rest: .... Duration: ....
   - Any sleep disturbance: ....
4. **Activities of daily living (ADLs)** (eating, grooming, dressing of elimination, locomotion), i.e:
   - Taking care and himself/herself: ....
   - Needs assistance: ....
   - Any problems with ADL: ....
   - Bladder frequency: .... Amount of urine: .... Character of urine: ....
   - Bowel condition: .... Amount of stool: .... Character of stool: ....
5. **Instrumental ADL (IADL)** (food preparation, shopping, transportation, housekeeping, laundry, ability to use telephone, handle finance, manage medication).

   Any problem with IADLs: ....
6. **Recreational and habits:**
   - Exercise activity and tolerance (specify): ....
   - Habits (specify): ....

7. **Socioeconomic status:**
   - Family relationship: Satisfactory/Unsatisfactory (specify): ....
   - Marital relationship: Satisfactory/Unsatisfactory (specify): ....
   - Occupational status: Employed/Unemployed/Business: ....
     Any occupational hazards (specify): ....
   - Economical status: Individual income: .... Sources: ....
     Family income: .... Sources: ....

Family History of Illness

Here member of the family tree, family report how and brief note of any family member having/had any illness. Death due to any disease (i.e. heart disease, cancer, diabetes, hypertension), obesity, alcoholism, any congenital problem and mental health disorders.

Family status: Nuclear/Joint

Family tree

Index
□ - Male
○ - Female
⊘ - Patient

Family Composition

Name of the Family Members	Relationship with Patient	Age/ Sex	Educational Status	Occupational Status	Marital Status	Health Status

History of health problem/chronic illness (specify): ....

Environmental History (Student Should Include the Following)

1. **Physical:** Living arrangements (types of housing, neighborhood, presence of hazards)

   (Mention about the where the patient living-house and locality, own or rented, type of house, lighting, ventilation, facility for water supply, kitchen, bathroom, latrine, garbage disposal, drainage, etc. whether maintain cleanliness, safety to live, any hazards of housing, etc. factor influencing in health and illness)

   ....

   ....

   ....

2. **Spiritual:** Extent to which religion on part of life, religion beliefs related to perception of health and illness, religious practices.

   ....

   ....

3. **Interpersonal:**
   - Ethnic background (language spoken, customs and values held folk practices used to maintain health or to cure illness) ....

     ....
   - Family relationships (family structure, roles, communication pattern, supports system)
   - Friendships—quality of relationships.

     ....

     ....

     ....

Points to be Consider for Present Illness

....

....

....

....

....

....

Nursing Diagnosis (problems related to health and illness)

1.
2.
3.
4.
5.

CASE 2

HISTORY TAKING

(ē Guidelines to Report History Taking)

BIOGRAPHICAL DATA

Name of the Patient: ....

Name of the Father/Guardian/Husband: ....

Age: .... Date of Birth: .... Sex: ....

Marital Status: .... Education: .... Occupation: ....

Monthly Income: ....

Mother Tongue: .... Religion: .... Nationality: ....

Educational Status: ....

Date of Admission: .... IP No: .... MLC/OP No: ....

Address: ....

....

....

Medical Diagnosis: .... Doctor's Name: ....

Name of the Hospital: ....

Ward: .... Bed Number: ....

Date of Data Collection: ....

Present History of Illness (Medical Surgical)

Give brief notes of onset of symptoms, their frequency, exact location of distress, character of complaints, e.g. intensity of pain, quality of sputum, emesis or discharge, etc.

For example: ....

....

....

....

....

....

....

....

....

Past History of Illness (Medical Surgical)

Mention brief note of history of childhood illnesses, childhood immunization, allergies, accidental injuries, hospitalization of serious illness, treatment given, complications and medication prescribed if anything that are in relevant to present health and disease.

....

....

....

Personal History

1. **Habits:** Substance use and abuse (i.e. tobacco, alcohol, coffee, tea, illicit or recreational drug, etc.) such as smoking, tobacco chewing, drug addiction (if present daily/occasionally, duration of use, exercises and yoga, etc.

   For example: Smoking: Yes/No: .... Per day: .... No. of years: ....
   Tobacco chewing: ....
   Alcohol: .... Drug addict (specify): ....
   ....
   ....

2. **Diet:** Members about typical diet, vegetarian and non-vegetarian/pattern of taking of meals:
   - Vegetarian: .... No of meals per day: ....
   - Any allergic to any food items: ....
3. **Sleep and rest pattern:**
   - Timing of sleep: .... Duration: ....
   - Timing of rest: .... Duration: ....
   - Any sleep disturbance: ....
4. **Activities of daily living (ADLs)** (eating, grooming, dressing of elimination, locomotion), i.e:
   - Taking care and himself/herself: ....
   - Needs assistance: ....
   - Any problems with ADL: ....
   - Bladder frequency: .... Amount of urine: .... Character of urine: ....
   - Bowel condition: .... Amount of stool: .... Character of stool: ....
5. **Instrumental ADL (IADL)** (food preparation, shopping, transportation, housekeeping, laundry, ability to use telephone, handle finance, manage medication).

   Any problem with IADLs: ....
6. **Recreational and habits:**
   - Exercise activity and tolerance (specify): ....
   - Habits (specify): ....

7. **Socioeconomic status:**
   - Family relationship: Satisfactory/Unsatisfactory (specify): ....
   - Marital relationship: Satisfactory/Unsatisfactory (specify): ....
   - Occupational status: Employed/Unemployed/Business: ....
     Any occupational hazards (specify): ....
   - Economical status: Individual income: .... Sources: ....
     Family income: .... Sources: ....

Family History of Illness

Here member of the family tree, family report how and brief note of any family member having/had any illness. Death due to any disease (i.e. heart disease, cancer, diabetes, hypertension), obesity, alcoholism, any congenital problem and mental health disorders.

Family status: Nuclear/Joint

Family tree

Index
□ - Male
○ - Female
⃠ - Patient

Family Composition

Name of the Family Members	Relationship with Patient	Age/ Sex	Educational Status	Occupational Status	Marital Status	Health Status

History of health problem/chronic illness (specify): ....

Environmental History (Student Should Include the Following)

1. **Physical:** Living arrangements (types of housing, neighborhood, presence of hazards)

   (Mention about the where the patient living-house and locality, own or rented, type of house, lighting, ventilation, facility for water supply, kitchen, bathroom, latrine, garbage disposal, drainage, etc. whether maintain cleanliness, safety to live, any hazards of housing, etc. factor influencing in health and illness)

   ....

   ....

   ....

2. **Spiritual:** Extent to which religion on part of life, religion beliefs related to perception of health and illness, religious practices.

   ....

   ....

3. **Interpersonal:**
   - Ethnic background (language spoken, customs and values held folk practices used to maintain health or to cure illness) ....

     ....
   - Family relationships (family structure, roles, communication pattern, supports system)
   - Friendships—quality of relationships.

     ....

     ....

     ....

Points to be Consider for Present Illness

....

....

....

....

....

....

Nursing Diagnosis (problems related to health and illness)

1.
2.
3.
4.
5.

CASE 3

HISTORY TAKING

(ē Guidelines to Report History Taking)

BIOGRAPHICAL DATA

Name of the Patient: ....

Name of the Father/Guardian/Husband: ....

Age: .... Date of Birth: .... Sex: ....

Marital Status: .... Education: .... Occupation: ....

Monthly Income: ....

Mother Tongue: .... Religion: .... Nationality: ....

Educational Status: ....

Date of Admission: .... IP No: .... MLC/OP No: ....

Address: ....

....

....

Medical Diagnosis: .... Doctor's Name: ....

Name of the Hospital: ....

Ward: .... Bed Number: ....

Date of Data Collection: ....

Present History of Illness (Medical Surgical)

Give brief notes of onset of symptoms, their frequency, exact location of distress, character of complaints, e.g. intensity of pain, quality of sputum, emesis or discharge, etc.

For example: ....

....

....

....

....

....

....

....

....

Past History of Illness (Medical Surgical)

Mention brief note of history of childhood illnesses, childhood immunization, allergies, accidental injuries, hospitalization of serious illness, treatment given, complications and medication prescribed if anything that are in relevant to present health and disease.

....

....

....

Personal History

1. **Habits:** Substance use and abuse (i.e. tobacco, alcohol, coffee, tea, illicit or recreational drug, etc.) such as smoking, tobacco chewing, drug addiction (if present daily/occasionally, duration of use, exercises and yoga, etc.

   For example: Smoking: Yes/No: .... Per day: .... No. of years: ....

   Tobacco chewing: ....

   Alcohol: .... Drug addict (specify): ....

   ....

   ....

2. **Diet:** Members about typical diet, vegetarian and non-vegetarian/pattern of taking of meals:
   - Vegetarian: .... No of meals per day: ....
   - Any allergic to any food items: ....
3. **Sleep and rest pattern:**
   - Timing of sleep: .... Duration: ....
   - Timing of rest: .... Duration: ....
   - Any sleep disturbance: ....
4. **Activities of daily living (ADLs)** (eating, grooming, dressing of elimination, locomotion), i.e:
   - Taking care and himself/herself: ....
   - Needs assistance: ....
   - Any problems with ADL: ....
   - Bladder frequency: .... Amount of urine: .... Character of urine: ....
   - Bowel condition: .... Amount of stool: .... Character of stool: ....
5. **Instrumental ADL (IADL)** (food preparation, shopping, transportation, housekeeping, laundry, ability to use telephone, handle finance, manage medication).

   Any problem with IADLs: ....

6. **Recreational and habits:**
   - Exercise activity and tolerance (specify): ....
   - Habits (specify): ....

7. **Socioeconomic status:**
   - Family relationship: Satisfactory/Unsatisfactory (specify): ....
   - Marital relationship: Satisfactory/Unsatisfactory (specify): ....
   - Occupational status: Employed/Unemployed/Business: ....
     Any occupational hazards (specify): ....
   - Economical status: Individual income: .... Sources: ....
     Family income: .... Sources: ....

Family History of Illness

Here member of the family tree, family report how and brief note of any family member having/had any illness. Death due to any disease (i.e. heart disease, cancer, diabetes, hypertension), obesity, alcoholism, any congenital problem and mental health disorders.

Family status: Nuclear/Joint

Family tree

Index
□ - Male
○ - Female
⊘ - Patient

Family Composition

Name of the Family Members	Relationship with Patient	Age/ Sex	Educational Status	Occupational Status	Marital Status	Health Status

History of health problem/chronic illness (specify): ....

Environmental History (Student Should Include the Following)

1. **Physical:** Living arrangements (types of housing, neighborhood, presence of hazards)

   (Mention about the where the patient living-house and locality, own or rented, type of house, lighting, ventilation, facility for water supply, kitchen, bathroom, latrine, garbage disposal, drainage, etc. whether maintain cleanliness, safety to live, any hazards of housing, etc. factor influencing in health and illness)

   ....

   ....

   ....

2. **Spiritual:** Extent to which religion on part of life, religion beliefs related to perception of health and illness, religious practices.

   ....

   ....

3. **Interpersonal:**
   - Ethnic background (language spoken, customs and values held folk practices used to maintain health or to cure illness) ....

     ....
   - Family relationships (family structure, roles, communication pattern, supports system)
   - Friendships—quality of relationships.

     ....

     ....

     ....

Points to be Consider for Present Illness

....

....

....

....

....

....

Nursing Diagnosis (problems related to health and illness)

1.
2.
3.
4.
5.

CASE 4

HISTORY TAKING

(ē Guidelines to Report History Taking)

BIOGRAPHICAL DATA

Name of the Patient: ....

Name of the Father/Guardian/Husband: ....

Age: .... Date of Birth: .... Sex: ....

Marital Status: .... Education: .... Occupation: ....

Monthly Income: ....

Mother Tongue: .... Religion: .... Nationality: ....

Educational Status: ....

Date of Admission: .... IP No: .... MLC/OP No: ....

Address: ....

....

....

Medical Diagnosis: .... Doctor's Name: ....

Name of the Hospital: ....

Ward: .... Bed Number: ....

Date of Data Collection: ....

Present History of Illness (Medical Surgical)

Give brief notes of onset of symptoms, their frequency, exact location of distress, character of complaints, e.g. intensity of pain, quality of sputum, emesis or discharge, etc.

For example: ....

....

....

....

....

....

....

....

....

Past History of Illness (Medical Surgical)

Mention brief note of history of childhood illnesses, childhood immunization, allergies, accidental injuries, hospitalization of serious illness, treatment given, complications and medication prescribed if anything that are in relevant to present health and disease.

....

....

....

Personal History

1. **Habits:** Substance use and abuse (i.e. tobacco, alcohol, coffee, tea, illicit or recreational drug, etc.) such as smoking, tobacco chewing, drug addiction (if present daily/occasionally, duration of use, exercises and yoga, etc.

   For example: Smoking: Yes/No: .... Per day: .... No. of years: ....

   Tobacco chewing: ....

   Alcohol: .... Drug addict (specify): ....

   ....

   ....

2. **Diet:** Members about typical diet, vegetarian and non-vegetarian/pattern of taking of meals:
   - Vegetarian: .... No of meals per day: ....
   - Any allergic to any food items: ....

3. **Sleep and rest pattern:**
   - Timing of sleep: .... Duration: ....
   - Timing of rest: .... Duration: ....
   - Any sleep disturbance: ....

4. **Activities of daily living (ADLs)** (eating, grooming, dressing of elimination, locomotion), i.e:
   - Taking care and himself/herself: ....
   - Needs assistance: ....
   - Any problems with ADL: ....
   - Bladder frequency: .... Amount of urine: .... Character of urine: ....
   - Bowel condition: .... Amount of stool: .... Character of stool: ....

5. **Instrumental ADL (IADL)** (food preparation, shopping, transportation, housekeeping, laundry, ability to use telephone, handle finance, manage medication).

   Any problem with IADLs: ....

6. **Recreational and habits:**
   - Exercise activity and tolerance (specify): ....
   - Habits (specify): ....

7. **Socioeconomic status:**
   - Family relationship: Satisfactory/Unsatisfactory (specify): ....
   - Marital relationship: Satisfactory/Unsatisfactory (specify): ....
   - Occupational status: Employed/Unemployed/Business: ....

     Any occupational hazards (specify): ....
   - Economical status: Individual income: .... Sources: ....

     Family income: .... Sources: ....

Family History of Illness

Here member of the family tree, family report how and brief note of any family member having/had any illness. Death due to any disease (i.e. heart disease, cancer, diabetes, hypertension), obesity, alcoholism, any congenital problem and mental health disorders.

Family status: Nuclear/Joint

Family tree

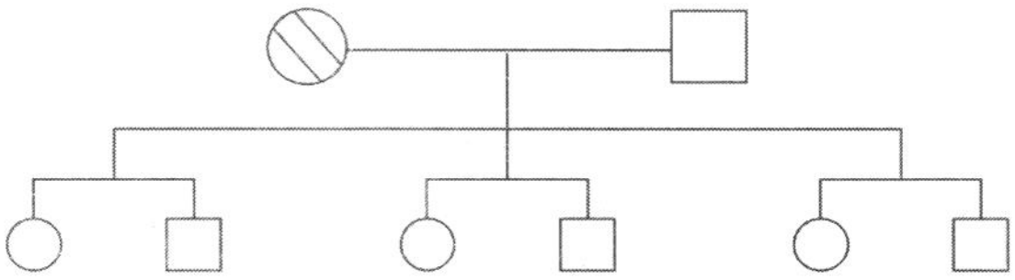

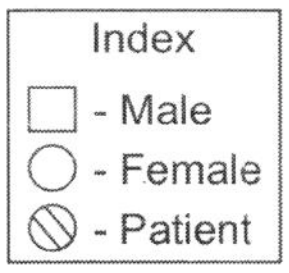

Index
- Male
- Female
- Patient

Family Composition

Name of the Family Members	Relationship with Patient	Age/ Sex	Educational Status	Occupational Status	Marital Status	Health Status

History of health problem/chronic illness (specify): ....

Environmental History (Student Should Include the Following)

1. **Physical:** Living arrangements (types of housing, neighborhood, presence of hazards)

   (Mention about the where the patient living-house and locality, own or rented, type of house, lighting, ventilation, facility for water supply, kitchen, bathroom, latrine, garbage disposal, drainage, etc. whether maintain cleanliness, safety to live, any hazards of housing, etc. factor influencing in health and illness)

   ....

   ....

   ....

2. **Spiritual:** Extent to which religion on part of life, religion beliefs related to perception of health and illness, religious practices.

   ....

   ....

3. **Interpersonal:**
   - Ethnic background (language spoken, customs and values held folk practices used to maintain health or to cure illness) ....

     ....
   - Family relationships (family structure, roles, communication pattern, supports system)
   - Friendships—quality of relationships.

     ....

     ....

     ....

Points to be Consider for Present Illness

....

....

....

....

....

....

Nursing Diagnosis (problems related to health and illness)

1.
2.
3.
4.
5.

CASE 5

HISTORY TAKING

(ē Guidelines to Report History Taking)

BIOGRAPHICAL DATA

Name of the Patient: ....

Name of the Father/Guardian/Husband: ....

Age: .... Date of Birth: .... Sex: ....

Marital Status: .... Education: .... Occupation: ....

Monthly Income: ....

Mother Tongue: .... Religion: .... Nationality: ....

Educational Status: ....

Date of Admission: .... IP No: .... MLC/OP No: ....

Address: ....

....

....

Medical Diagnosis: .... Doctor's Name: ....

Name of the Hospital: ....

Ward: .... Bed Number: ....

Date of Data Collection: ....

Present History of Illness (Medical Surgical)

Give brief notes of onset of symptoms, their frequency, exact location of distress, character of complaints, e.g. intensity of pain, quality of sputum, emesis or discharge, etc.

For example: ....

....

....

....

....

....

....

....

....

Past History of Illness (Medical Surgical)

Mention brief note of history of childhood illnesses, childhood immunization, allergies, accidental injuries, hospitalization of serious illness, treatment given, complications and medication prescribed if anything that are in relevant to present health and disease.

....

....

....

Personal History

1. **Habits:** Substance use and abuse (i.e. tobacco, alcohol, coffee, tea, illicit or recreational drug, etc.) such as smoking, tobacco chewing, drug addiction (if present daily/occasionally, duration of use, exercises and yoga, etc.

   For example: Smoking: Yes/No: .... Per day: .... No. of years: ....

   Tobacco chewing: ....

   Alcohol: .... Drug addict (specify): ....

   ....

   ....

2. **Diet:** Members about typical diet, vegetarian and non-vegetarian/pattern of taking of meals:
   - Vegetarian: .... No of meals per day: ....
   - Any allergic to any food items: ....

3. **Sleep and rest pattern:**
   - Timing of sleep: .... Duration: ....
   - Timing of rest: .... Duration: ....
   - Any sleep disturbance: ....

4. **Activities of daily living (ADLs)** (eating, grooming, dressing of elimination, locomotion), i.e:
   - Taking care and himself/herself: ....
   - Needs assistance: ....
   - Any problems with ADL: ....
   - Bladder frequency: .... Amount of urine: .... Character of urine: ....
   - Bowel condition: .... Amount of stool: .... Character of stool: ....

5. **Instrumental ADL (IADL)** (food preparation, shopping, transportation, housekeeping, laundry, ability to use telephone, handle finance, manage medication).

   Any problem with IADLs: ....

6. **Recreational and habits:**
   - Exercise activity and tolerance (specify): ....
   - Habits (specify): ....

7. **Socioeconomic status:**
   - Family relationship: Satisfactory/Unsatisfactory (specify): ....
   - Marital relationship: Satisfactory/Unsatisfactory (specify): ....
   - Occupational status: Employed/Unemployed/Business: ....
     Any occupational hazards (specify): ....
   - Economical status: Individual income: .... Sources: ....
     Family income: .... Sources: ....

Family History of Illness

Here member of the family tree, family report how and brief note of any family member having/had any illness. Death due to any disease (i.e. heart disease, cancer, diabetes, hypertension), obesity, alcoholism, any congenital problem and mental health disorders.

Family status: Nuclear/Joint

Family tree

Index
- Male
- Female
- Patient

Family Composition

Name of the Family Members	Relationship with Patient	Age/ Sex	Educational Status	Occupational Status	Marital Status	Health Status

History of health problem/chronic illness (specify): ....

Environmental History (Student Should Include the Following)

1. **Physical:** Living arrangements (types of housing, neighborhood, presence of hazards)

   (Mention about the where the patient living-house and locality, own or rented, type of house, lighting, ventilation, facility for water supply, kitchen, bathroom, latrine, garbage disposal, drainage, etc. whether maintain cleanliness, safety to live, any hazards of housing, etc. factor influencing in health and illness)

   ....

   ....

   ....

2. **Spiritual:** Extent to which religion on part of life, religion beliefs related to perception of health and illness, religious practices.

   ....

   ....

3. **Interpersonal:**
   - Ethnic background (language spoken, customs and values held folk practices used to maintain health or to cure illness) ....

     ....
   - Family relationships (family structure, roles, communication pattern, supports system)
   - Friendships—quality of relationships.

     ....

     ....

     ....

Points to be Consider for Present Illness

....

....

....

....

....

....

Nursing Diagnosis (problems related to health and illness)

1.
2.
3.
4.
5.

SECTION II

PHYSICAL EXAMINATION

Guidelines to Report Physical Examination

Note: Students are instructed to use following descriptive terminology suggested for documentation of physical examination and write suitable terms in the space provided.

General Appearance

- **Level of consciousness:** Conscious/Unconscious/Semiconscious/Coma ....
- **Orientation:** To place/To person/To time ....
- **Activity:** Active/Dull/Lethargic ....
- **Body built:** Mild/Moderate/Thin/Obese/Emaciated/Flabby ....
- **Height:** ....
- **Weight:** ....,weight appropriate to height ....
- **Mid upper arm circumference:** ....
- **General grooming:** Clean/Hair combed/Make up ....
- **Position/Posturing:** Supine/Prone/Rigid/Opisthotonos/Erect/Slumped ....
- **Facial expression:** Smiling/Frowning/Blank/Apathetic ....
- **Body language:** Eye contact/No eye contact/Arms folded over chest ....
- **Other observations:** Restless/Fidgeting/Lying quietly/Listless/Trembling/Tense ....

Skin Inspection and Palpation (Integumentary System)

- **Color and vascularity:**
  - Pink/Tan/Brown/Flushed/Jaundiced ....
  - Dark brown/Grayish/Pasty/Yellowish ....
- **Turgor and mobility:** Elastic/Nonelastic/Tenting/Wrinkles/Edematous tight ....
- **Temperature and moisture:**
  - Cold/Cool/Warm/Hot/Feverish/Sweating ....
  - Moist/Dry/Clammy/Oily/Diaphoresis ....
- **Texture:** Smooth/Rough/Fine/Thick/Coarse/Scaly/Puffy ....
- **Nails:**
  - Clean manicured/Smooth/Rough/Yellowing/Paronychia ....
  - Dry/Hard/Brittle/Splitting/Cracking/Angle of nail bed/Clubbing/Curved/Flat/Thick ....

- **Nail beds and lunulae:** Pale/Pink/Cyanotic/Red/Shape of lunula/Blanching/Spooning ....
- **Body hair growth:** Color/Thick/Thin/Coarse/Fine/Hirsutism ....
- **Skin integrity:**
  - Intact/Not intact/Birth marks/Moles/Scars ....
  - Lesions/Fissures/Acules/Papules/Pustules/Nodules/Cysts/Carbuncle/Wheals/Erythema/Excoriation/Desquamation/Abrasions/Cherry angiomas/Senile lentigines/Senile purpura/Insect Bites/Crusts/Warts/Pimples/Black heads/Bleeding/Drainage/Scaly/Ulcers/Lacerations ....

Head Inspection and Palpation

- **Shape:** Round/Oval/Square/Pointed/Normocephalic ....
- **Face:**
  - Oval/Heart shaped/Pear/Long square/Symmetrical/Round/Thin/High cheekbones ....
  - Sensations [trigeminal cranial nerve (CN) V]: Sensation on three branches/Clenched teeth ....
- **Facial (CN VII):** Facial expressions/Smiles ....
- **Hair:**
  - Color and growth coarse/Fine/Thin/Sparse/Alopecia ....
  - Long/Short/Curly/Straight/Permed/Glossy/Shiny/Greasy/Dry/Brittle/Stringy/Frizzy ....
- **Condition of scalp:** Clean/Scaly/Dandruff/Rashes/Sores/Drainage ....
- **Masses and lumps:** Location, size, shape ....
- **Facial puffiness:** Present/Absent ....

Eyes Inspection and Palpation

- **Eyebrows:** Color, shape alignment/Straight/Curved/Thick/Thin/Scaly/Plucked/Sparse ....
- **Eyelashes:** Long/Short/Curved/Artificial ....
- **Eyelids:** Dark/Swollen/Inflamed/Discharge/Stye/Ptosis/Entropion/Ectropion/Lid lag/Xanthomas open and close simultaneously ....
- **Shape and appearance:** Almond/Rounded/Squinty/Prominent/Strabismus/Nystagmus/Exophthalmic/Sunken/Bright/Clear/Dull/Tearing/Discharge/Exotropia/Esotropia ....
- **Sclera:** White/Cream/Yellowish/Jaundiced/Infected/Pterygium ....
- **Conjunctiva:** Pale pink/Pink/Red/Inflamed/Swelling/Nodules ....
- **Iris:** Color and shape, round/Flat/Coloboma/Arcus senilis ....
- **Cornea:** Clear/Milky/Opaque/Cloudy ....
- **Pupils (oculomotor-CN III)—pupils equal, round, reactive to light accommodation (PERRLA):**
  - Size and shape (round/not round) ....
  - Describe equality; symmetrical/Anisocoria/Right larger than left/Left larger than right/Convergence/Reaction to light and accommodation/Consensual reaction/Extraocular movements/Trochlear/Abducens/Dilated/Constricted/Unequal/Fixed ....

- **Lacrimal glands:** Tender/Nontender/Inflamed/Swollen/Tearing ....
- **Visual field:** Intact/Not intact ....
- **Vision:** Reads/Reports ....
- **Use of glasses:** Glasses/Contact lenses/Prosthesis ....

Ears Inspection and Palpation

- **Pinnae:** Size and shape—large/Small/In proportion to face/Protruding oval/Large lobes/Small lobes/Symmetrical/Right larger than left/Left larger than right/Pinnae irregular/Color/Skin intact/Redness/Swelling/Tophi/Cauliflower ear/Furuncles/Darwin's tubercle ....
- **Level in relation to eyes:** Top of pinnae level with outer canthus of eyes/Top of pinnae lower than outer canthus of eyes/Top of pinnae higher than outer canthus of eyes ....
- **Canal:** Clean/Discharge/Redness/Foreign object ....
- **Cilia:** Present/Absent ....
- **Cerumen:** Present/Absent/Color/Consistency ....
- **Tympanic membrane:** Color/Pearly white/Red/Inflamed/Cone of light/Land marks/Scarring/Bubbles/Fluid level ....
- **Hearing (audition- CN VIII):**
  - Right present/Absent ....
  - Left present/Absent ....
- **Tuning fork test:** Listen/Not listen ....
- **Weber test:** Lateralizes equally to left/right side ....
- **Rinne test:** Air conduction bone conduction 2:1 ....
- **Hearing aid:** Yes/No, right/left ....

Nose and Sinuses Inspection and Palpation

- **Size and shape:**
  - Long/Short/Large/Small ....
  - In proportion to face/flat/broad/broad based/thick/thin/enlarged/nares symmetrical/asymmetrical/pointed/swollen/bulbous/flaring of nostrils ....
- **Nasal septum:**
  - Midline/Deviated to right or left/Perforated ....
- **Nasal mucosa and turbinate:**
  - Pink/Pale/Bluish/Red/Dry ....
  - Moist/Discharge/Cilia present/Absent/Rhinitis/Epistaxis/Polyps ....
- **Patency of nares:** Right patent/Partial obstruction ....

- **Olfactory(CN I):** Correctly identifies odors ....
- **Sinuses:** Tender/Nontender/Transillumination ....

Mouth and Pharynx Inspection (Oral Cavity Examination)

- **Lips:**
  - Color: Pink/Red/Pale/Tam/Cyanotic ....
  - Shape: Thin/Thick/Enlarged/Swollen/Symmetrical/Asymmetrical/Drooping left side/Drooping right side ....
  - Condition: Soft/Smooth/Dry/Cracked/Fissured/Blisters/Lesions ....
- **Teeth:**
  - Color and condition: White/Yellow/Grayish/Spotted/Stained/Darkened/Pitting/Notched/Straight/Crooked/Protruding/Separated/Crowded/Irregular/Broken/Notching/Peglike/Loose/Dull/Bright/Dentulous/Malocclusion ....
- **Dental caries and fillings:** Number and location ....
- **Dental hygiene:** Clean/Not clean, etc. ....
- **Breathe odor:**
  - Sweet/Odorless/Halitosis ....
  - Musty/Acetone/Foul/Fetid/Odor of drugs or food/Hot/Sour/Alcohol ....
- **Gums:**
  - Pink/Firm/Swollen/Bleeding ....
  - Sensitive/Gingivitis/Hypertrophy ....
  - Nodules/Irritated/Receding/Moist/Ulcerated/Dry/Shrunken/Blistered/Spongy ....
- **Facial and glossopharyngeal (CN VII and IX):** identifies taste ....
- **Tongue:**
  - Thick/Thin/Pink/Pale/Bluish ....
  - Macroglossia/Microglossia/Glossitis/Geographic/Red/Swollen/Clean/Fissured/Coated/Moist/Dry/Cracked/Glistening/Papillae ....
- **Hypoglossal (CN XII):** Tongue movement; symmetry/lateral/fasciculation ....
- **Mucosa:**
  - Color/Leukoplakia/Dry/Moist ....
  - Intact/Not intact/Masses/Chancre ....
- **Palate:** Moist/Dry/Color/Intact/Not intact ....
- **Uvula:** Color/Midline ....
- **Pharynx:** Color/Petechiae/Injected/Beefy/Dysphagia ....
- **Tonsils:** Present/Absent/Crypt/Beefy ....
- **Temporomandibular joint:** Fully mobile symmetry/Tenderness/Crepitus ....

Neck Inspection and Palpation

- **Appearance:** Long/Short/Thick/Thin/Masses/Size and shape; symmetrical/not symmetrical ....
- **Thyroid:** Palpable/Nodules/Tender ....
- **Trachea:** Midline/Deviated to right/left ....
- **Lymph nodes:** Occipito preauricular/postauricular/submental/submaxillary/tonsillar/anterior cervical/posterior cervical/superficial cervical/deep cervical/nonpalpable/tender/lymphadenopathy/shotty/hard/firm ....

Thorax and Lung Examination (Respiratory System)

- **Respiratory rate:**
  - Tachypnea/Eupnoea/Apnea/Bradypnea/Orthopnea/Labored/Stertorous ....
  - Rhythm: Regular/Irregular/Inspiration time greater than expiration time/Expiration time is greater than inspiration time/Spasmodic/gasping/Orthopneic/Deep/Eupneic/Shallow/Accessory muscles used/Pigeon chest/Barrel chest/Abdominal chest breather/Funnel chest/Lesions ....
- **Thoracic cage shape:** Barrel chest/Scoliosis/Kyphosis/Normal ....
- **Configuration:** Pectus excavatum/Pectus carinatum/Normal ....
- **Skin color and condition:** Normal/Cyanosis/Pallor ....
- **Chest examination:** Symmetric/Asymmetric ....
- **Posterior thorax:** Tenderness/Masses/Respiratory excursion; symmetrical/asymmetrical/no respiratory movements on right/left side/Subcutaneous emphysema/Crepitus/Fremitus/Estimation of level of diaphragm/Spine alignment/Costovertebral angle (CVA) tenderness/Resonance/Dull/Hyper resonance
- **Percussion on lung field:** Clear/Not clear ....
- **Diaphragmatic exertion:** Dull/Normal ....
- **Lung auscultation:** Vesicular/Bronchovesicular/Bronchial/Whispered pectoriloquy/Adventitious sounds/Rales/Rhonchi/Wheezes/Crackles/Rub/Egophony/Bronchophony ....
- **Breath sound:** Vesicular/Bronchovesicular ....
- **Respiratory pattern:** Normal/Abnormal (specify) ....

Breasts and Axillae Inspection and Palpation

- **Male breasts:** Lumps/Swelling/Gynecomastia ....
- **Female breasts:**
  - Symmetry/Pain/Lump/Discharge ....
  - Trauma/Abnormalities/Surgery, etc. ....
- **Nipples:** Present/Absent/Circular/Symmetrical/Asymmetrical/Inverted/Everted/Pale/Brown/Extra nipples/Discharge/Deviation/Supernumerary ....
- **Axilla:** Shaved/Unshaved/Odor/Lump masses ....

Cardiovascular Examination

- **Heart:** Precordial bulge/Abnormal palpitations/Point of maximal impulse (PMI)/Thrills/S1 loudest at apex/S2 loudest at base/S3/S4/Splits/Clicks/Snap/Rub/Gallop ....
- **Heart sounds:** S1, S2 heard/Abnormalities ....
- **Murmurs:** Systolic/Diastolic/Holosystolic/Harsh/Soft/Blowing/Rumbling/High pitch/Low pitch/Medium pitch ....
- **Carotid pulse:** Volume/Rhythm ....
- **Apical pulse:** Tachycardia/Bradycardia/Pounding forceful, Weak/Moderate/Regular/Irregular ....
- **Peripheral pulses:** Volume/Rhythm/Symmetry ....
- **Blood pressure:** .... **Pulse rate:** ....

Abdominal Examination

- **Contour:**
  - Irregular/Protruding/Enlarged/Distended ....
  - Scaphoid/Concave/Sunken/Flabby/Firm/Flat/Flaccid ....
- **Skin:** Color; Intact/Not intact/Shiny/Smooth/Scars/Lesions/Striae/Umbilicus ....
- **Bowel sounds:** Present/Absent/Hyperactive/High-pitched tickling/Gurgles/Borborygmus ....
- **On percussion:** Tympanic/Dull/Flat (describe where) ascites/Fluid collection ....
- **Palpation:** Splenomegaly/Hepatomegaly/Organomegaly/Masses/Aortic pulse/Diastasis recti/Tenderness/Bulges/Inguinal/Femoral hernia/Inguinal nodes ....

Musculoskeletal Examination

- **Back:** Shoulders level/Right shoulder higher than left/Left shoulder higher than right/Alignment/Lordosis/Scoliosis/Kyphosis ....
- **Vertebral column alignment:** Straight/Scoliosis/Lordosis/Kyphosis/Ankylosis ....
- **Joints:** Redness/Swelling/Deformities/Subluxation/Separation/Bogginess/Tenderness/Pain/Thickening/Nodules/Fluid/Bulging ....
- **Range of motion:**
  - Full/Limited/Fixed ....
  - Assess range of motion of neck, shoulders, elbows wrists, fingers, back, hips, knees, ankles, toes ....
- **Extremities:** Color/Symmetry/Variations/Temperature/Hot/Warm/Cool/Cold/Moist/Clammy/Dry, muscle tone descriptors are firm/Muscular/Flabby/Flaccid/Atrophy/Tremor ....
- **Lower extremities:** Symmetry, variations, prosthesis/varicose veins ....

Genitourinary and Rectum Inspection

- **Rectum:** Hemorrhoids/Inflammation/Fissures/Lesions/Skin tags/Excoriation/Swelling/Mucosal bulging/Rectocele ....
- **Female genitalia:**
  - Pubic hair distribution, color, nits/Lesions/Nodules ....
  - Varicosities/Swelling/Pigmentation/Dry/Moist/Shrivelled/Atrophy/Discharge/Odor/Asymmetry/Uterine prolapsed/Smegma/Rash ....
- **Male genitalia:** Pubic hair distribution, color, nits/circumcised/phimosis, hydrocele, epispadias, hypospadias, priapism, cryptorchidism, swelling, redness, chancre/cruising/rash/discharge/edema/scrotal sack rugated/atrophy ....

Neurological Examination

- **Describe:** Tics/Twitches/Paresthesia/Paralysis/Coordination ....
- **Gait:** Balanced/Shuffling/Unsteady/Ataxic/Parkinsonian/Swaying/Scissor/Spastic/Waddling/Staggering/Faltering/Slow/Difficult/Tottering/Propulsive ....
- **Accessory CN XI:** Shrugs shoulder/Symmetry ....
- **Reflex:** Report as present/absent ....
- **Coordination:** Report as to test done ....
- **Cranial nerves:** May be reported here ....

Mental Status Examination

- **Level of alertness:** Alert/Stuporous/Semicomatose ....
- **Orientation:**
  - Oriented to time, place, person ....
  - Confused/Disoriented ....
- **Memory:**
  - Recent memory ....
  - Long-term memory ....
- **Language and speech:**
  - Language ....
  - Speech, slow/Rapid/Slurred/Difficulty forming words/Aphasia ....
- **Responsiveness:**
  - Responds to verbal stimuli ....
  - Type of response slow/rapid ....

- **Knowledge test:** ....
- **Thinking:** ....
- **Judgment:** ....
- **Insight:** ....

Final Impression and Suspected Illness/Disease

....

....

....

....

....

CASE 1

PHYSICAL EXAMINATION

Name of the Patient: .... **Age:** .... **Sex:** ....

Educational Status: ....

Date of Admission: .... **IP No:** .... **MLC/OP No:** ....

Medical Diagnosis: ....

General Appearance

- Level of consciousness: ....
- Activity: ....
- Body built: ....
- Height: ....
- Weight: ....
- Mid-upper arm circumference: ....
- General grooming: ....
- Position/Posturing: ....
- Facial expression: ....
- Body language: ....
- Other observations: ....

Skin Inspection and Palpation

- Color and vascularity: ....
- Turgor and mobility: ....
- Temperature and moisture: ....
- Texture: ....
- Nails: ....
- Body hair growth: ....
- Skin integrity: ....
- Lesions: ....

Head Inspection and Palpation

- Shape: ....
- Face: ....
- Sensations (CN V): ....

- Facial (CN V): ....
- Hair: ....
- Condition of scalp: ....
- Masses and lumps: ....
- Facial puffiness: ....

Eyes Inspection and Palpation

- Eyebrows: ....
- Eyelashes: ....
- Eyelids: ....
- Shape and appearance: ....
- Sclera: ....
- Conjunctiva: ....
- Iris: ....
- Cornea: ....
- Pupils: ....
- Visual field: ....
- Vision: ....
- Use of glasses: ....

Ears Inspection and Palpation

- Pinnae: ....
- Level in relation to eyes: ....
- Canal: ....
- Cilia: ....
- Cerumen: ....
- Tympanic membrane: ....
- Hearing (audition-CN VIII): ....
- Tuning fork test: ....
- Weber test: ....
- Rinne test: ....
- Hearing aid: ....

Nose and Sinuses Inspection and Palpation

- Size and shape: ....
- Nasal septum: ....

- Nasal mucosa and turbinate: ....
- Patency of nares: ....
- Olfactory (CN I): ....
- Sinuses: ....

Mouth and Pharynx Inspection

- Lips: ....
- Teeth: ....
- Dental caries and fillings: ....
- Dental hygiene: ....
- Breath odor: ....
- Gums: ....
- Facial and glossopharyngeal (CN VII and IX): ....
- Tongue: ....
- Hypoglossal (CN XII): ....
- Mucosa: ....
- Palate: ....
- Uvula: ....
- Pharynx: ....
- Tonsils: ....
- Temporomandibular joint: ....

Neck Inspection and Palpation

- Appearance: ....
- Thyroid: ....
- Trachea: ....
- Lymph nodes: ....

Thorax and Lung Examination

- Respiratory rate: ....
- Thoracic cage shape: ....
- Configuration: ....
- Skin color and condition: ....
- Chest examination: ....
- Posterior thorax: ....

- Percussion on lung field: ....
- Diaphragmatic exertion: ....
- Lung auscultation: ....
- Breath sound: ....
- Respiratory pattern: ....

Breasts and Axillae Inspection and Palpation

- Male breasts: ....
- Female breasts: ....
- Nipples: ....
- Axilla: ....

Cardiovascular Examination

- Heart: ....
- Heart sounds: ....
- Murmurs: ....
- Carotid pulse: ....
- Apical pulse: ....
- Peripheral pulses: ....
- Blood pressure: .... Pulse rate: ....

Abdominal Examination

- Contour: ....
- Skin: ....
- Bowel sounds: ....
- On percussion: ....
- Palpation: ....

Musculoskeletal Examination

- Back: ....
- Vertebral column alignment: ....
- Joints: ....
- Range of motion: ....
- Extremities: ....
- Lower extremities: ....

Genitourinary and Rectum Inspection

- Rectum: ....
- Female genitalia: ....
- Male genitalia: ....

Neurological Examination

- Describe tics, twitches, paresthesia: ....
- Gait: ....
- Accessory (CN XI): ....
- Reflex: ....
- Coordination: ....
- Cranial nerves: ....

Mental Status Examination

- Level of alertness: ....
- Orientation: ....
- Memory: ....
- Language and speech: ....
- Responsiveness: ....
- Knowledge test: ....
- Thinking: ....
- Judgment: ....
- Insight: ....

Final Impression and Suspected Illness/Disease (States the Problem or Nursing Diagnosis)

....

....

....

....

....

CASE 2

PHYSICAL EXAMINATION

Name of the Patient: .... **Age:** .... **Sex:** ....

Educational Status: ....

Date of Admission: .... **IP No:** .... **MLC/OP No:** ....

Medical Diagnosis: ....

General Appearance

- Level of consciousness: ....
- Activity: ....
- Body built: ....
- Height: ....
- Weight: ....
- Mid-upper arm circumference: ....
- General grooming: ....
- Position/Posturing: ....
- Facial expression: ....
- Body language: ....
- Other observations: ....

Skin Inspection and Palpation

- Color and vascularity: ....
- Turgor and mobility: ....
- Temperature and moisture: ....
- Texture: ....
- Nails: ....
- Body hair growth: ....
- Skin integrity: ....
- Lesions: ....

Head Inspection and Palpation

- Shape: ....
- Face: ....
- Sensations (CN V): ....

- Facial (CN V): ....
- Hair: ....
- Condition of scalp: ....
- Masses and lumps: ....
- Facial puffiness: ....

Eyes Inspection and Palpation

- Eyebrows: ....
- Eyelashes: ....
- Eyelids: ....
- Shape and appearance: ....
- Sclera: ....
- Conjunctiva: ....
- Iris: ....
- Cornea: ....
- Pupils: ....
- Visual field: ....
- Vision: ....
- Use of glasses: ....

Ears Inspection and Palpation

- Pinnae: ....
- Level in relation to eyes: ....
- Canal: ....
- Cilia: ....
- Cerumen: ....
- Tympanic membrane: ....
- Hearing (audition-CN VIII): ....
- Tuning fork test: ....
- Weber test: ....
- Rinne test: ....
- Hearing aid: ....

Nose and Sinuses Inspection and Palpation

- Size and shape: ....
- Nasal septum: ....

- Nasal mucosa and turbinate: ....
- Patency of nares: ....
- Olfactory (CN I): ....
- Sinuses: ....

Mouth and Pharynx Inspection

- Lips: ....
- Teeth: ....
- Dental caries and fillings: ....
- Dental hygiene: ....
- Breath odor: ....
- Gums: ....
- Facial and glossopharyngeal (CN VII and IX): ....
- Tongue: ....
- Hypoglossal (CN XII): ....
- Mucosa: ....
- Palate: ....
- Uvula: ....
- Pharynx: ....
- Tonsils: ....
- Temporomandibular joint: ....

Neck Inspection and Palpation

- Appearance: ....
- Thyroid: ....
- Trachea: ....
- Lymph nodes: ....

Thorax and Lung Examination

- Respiratory rate: ....
- Thoracic cage shape: ....
- Configuration: ....
- Skin color and condition: ....
- Chest examination: ....
- Posterior thorax: ....

- Percussion on lung field: ....
- Diaphragmatic exertion: ....
- Lung auscultation: ....
- Breath sound: ....
- Respiratory pattern: ....

Breasts and Axillae Inspection and Palpation

- Male breasts: ....
- Female breasts: ....
- Nipples: ....
- Axilla: ....

Cardiovascular Examination

- Heart: ....
- Heart sounds: ....
- Murmurs: ....
- Carotid pulse: ....
- Apical pulse: ....
- Peripheral pulses: ....
- Blood pressure: .... Pulse rate: ....

Abdominal Examination

- Contour: ....
- Skin: ....
- Bowel sounds: ....
- On percussion: ....
- Palpation: ....

Musculoskeletal Examination

- Back: ....
- Vertebral column alignment: ....
- Joints: ....
- Range of motion: ....
- Extremities: ....
- Lower extremities: ....

Genitourinary and Rectum Inspection

- Rectum: ....
- Female genitalia: ....
- Male genitalia: ....

Neurological Examination

- Describe tics, twitches, paresthesia: ....
- Gait:..
- Accessory (CN XI): ....
- Reflex: ....
- Coordination: ....
- Cranial nerves: ....

Mental Status Examination

- Level of alertness: ....
- Orientation: ....
- Memory: ....
- Language and speech: ....
- Responsiveness: ....
- Knowledge test: ....
- Thinking: ....
- Judgment: ....
- Insight: ....

Final Impression and Suspected Illness/Disease (States the Problem or Nursing Diagnosis)

....

....

....

....

....

CASE 3

PHYSICAL EXAMINATION

Name of the Patient: .... **Age:** .... **Sex:** ....

Educational Status: ....

Date of Admission: .... **IP No:** .... **MLC/OP No:** ....

Medical Diagnosis: ....

General Appearance

- Level of consciousness: ....
- Activity: ....
- Body built: ....
- Height: ....
- Weight: ....
- Mid-upper arm circumference: ....
- General grooming: ....
- Position/Posturing: ....
- Facial expression: ....
- Body language: ....
- Other observations: ....

Skin Inspection and Palpation

- Color and vascularity: ....
- Turgor and mobility: ....
- Temperature and moisture: ....
- Texture: ....
- Nails: ....
- Body hair growth: ....
- Skin integrity: ....
- Lesions: ....

Head Inspection and Palpation

- Shape: ....
- Face: ....
- Sensations (CN V): ....

- Facial (CN V): ....
- Hair: ....
- Condition of scalp: ....
- Masses and lumps: ....
- Facial puffiness: ....

Eyes Inspection and Palpation

- Eyebrows: ....
- Eyelashes: ....
- Eyelids: ....
- Shape and appearance: ....
- Sclera: ....
- Conjunctiva: ....
- Iris: ....
- Cornea: ....
- Pupils: ....
- Visual field: ....
- Vision: ....
- Use of glasses: ....

Ears Inspection and Palpation

- Pinnae: ....
- Level in relation to eyes: ....
- Canal: ....
- Cilia: ....
- Cerumen: ....
- Tympanic membrane: ....
- Hearing (audition-CN VIII): ....
- Tuning fork test: ....
- Weber test: ....
- Rinne test: ....
- Hearing aid: ....

Nose and Sinuses Inspection and Palpation

- Size and shape: ....
- Nasal septum: ....

- Nasal mucosa and turbinate: ....
- Patency of nares: ....
- Olfactory (CN I): ....
- Sinuses: ....

Mouth and Pharynx Inspection

- Lips: ....
- Teeth: ....
- Dental caries and fillings: ....
- Dental hygiene: ....
- Breath odor: ....
- Gums: ....
- Facial and glossopharyngeal (CN VII and IX): ....
- Tongue: ....
- Hypoglossal (CN XII): ....
- Mucosa: ....
- Palate: ....
- Uvula: ....
- Pharynx: ....
- Tonsils: ....
- Temporomandibular joint: ....

Neck Inspection and Palpation

- Appearance: ....
- Thyroid: ....
- Trachea: ....
- Lymph nodes: ....

Thorax and Lung Examination

- Respiratory rate: ....
- Thoracic cage shape: ....
- Configuration: ....
- Skin color and condition: ....
- Chest examination: ....
- Posterior thorax: ....

- Percussion on lung field:
- Diaphragmatic exertion:
- Lung auscultation:
- Breath sound:
- Respiratory pattern:

Breasts and Axillae Inspection and Palpation

- Male breasts:
- Female breasts:
- Nipples:
- Axilla:

Cardiovascular Examination

- Heart:
- Heart sounds:
- Murmurs:
- Carotid pulse:
- Apical pulse:
- Peripheral pulses:
- Blood pressure: Pulse rate:

Abdominal Examination

- Contour:
- Skin:
- Bowel sounds:
- On percussion:
- Palpation:

Musculoskeletal Examination

- Back:
- Vertebral column alignment:
- Joints:
- Range of motion:
- Extremities:
- Lower extremities:

Genitourinary and Rectum Inspection

- Rectum: ....
- Female genitalia: ....
- Male genitalia: ....

Neurological Examination

- Describe tics, twitches, paresthesia: ....
- Gait: ....
- Accessory (CN XI): ....
- Reflex: ....
- Coordination: ....
- Cranial nerves: ....

Mental Status Examination

- Level of alertness: ....
- Orientation: ....
- Memory: ....
- Language and speech: ....
- Responsiveness: ....
- Knowledge test: ....
- Thinking: ....
- Judgment: ....
- Insight: ....

Final Impression and Suspected Illness/Disease (States the Problem or Nursing Diagnosis)

....

....

....

....

....

CASE 4

PHYSICAL EXAMINATION

Name of the Patient: .... **Age:** .... **Sex:** ....

Educational Status: ....

Date of Admission: .... **IP No:** .... **MLC/OP No:** ....

Medical Diagnosis: ....

General Appearance

- Level of consciousness: ....
- Activity: ....
- Body built: ....
- Height: ....
- Weight: ....
- Mid-upper arm circumference: ....
- General grooming: ....
- Position/Posturing: ....
- Facial expression: ....
- Body language: ....
- Other observations: ....

Skin Inspection and Palpation

- Color and vascularity: ....
- Turgor and mobility: ....
- Temperature and moisture: ....
- Texture: ....
- Nails: ....
- Body hair growth: ....
- Skin integrity: ....
- Lesions: ....

Head Inspection and Palpation

- Shape: ....
- Face: ....
- Sensations (CN V): ....

- Facial (CN V): ....
- Hair: ....
- Condition of scalp: ....
- Masses and lumps: ....
- Facial puffiness: ....

Eyes Inspection and Palpation

- Eyebrows: ....
- Eyelashes: ....
- Eyelids: ....
- Shape and appearance: ....
- Sclera: ....
- Conjunctiva: ....
- Iris: ....
- Cornea: ....
- Pupils: ....
- Visual field: ....
- Vision: ....
- Use of glasses: ....

Ears Inspection and Palpation

- Pinnae: ....
- Level in relation to eyes: ....
- Canal: ....
- Cilia: ....
- Cerumen: ....
- Tympanic membrane: ....
- Hearing (audition-CN VIII): ....
- Tuning fork test: ....
- Weber test: ....
- Rinne test: ....
- Hearing aid: ....

Nose and Sinuses Inspection and Palpation

- Size and shape: ....
- Nasal septum: ....

- Nasal mucosa and turbinate: ....
- Patency of nares: ....
- Olfactory (CN I): ....
- Sinuses: ....

Mouth and Pharynx Inspection

- Lips: ....
- Teeth: ....
- Dental caries and fillings: ....
- Dental hygiene: ....
- Breath odor: ....
- Gums: ....
- Facial and glossopharyngeal (CN VII and IX): ....
- Tongue: ....
- Hypoglossal (CN XII): ....
- Mucosa: ....
- Palate: ....
- Uvula: ....
- Pharynx: ....
- Tonsils: ....
- Temporomandibular joint: ....

Neck Inspection and Palpation

- Appearance: ....
- Thyroid: ....
- Trachea: ....
- Lymph nodes: ....

Thorax and Lung Examination

- Respiratory rate: ....
- Thoracic cage shape: ....
- Configuration: ....
- Skin color and condition: ....
- Chest examination: ....
- Posterior thorax: ....

- Percussion on lung field: ....
- Diaphragmatic exertion: ....
- Lung auscultation: ....
- Breath sound: ....
- Respiratory pattern: ....

Breasts and Axillae Inspection and Palpation

- Male breasts: ....
- Female breasts: ....
- Nipples: ....
- Axilla: ....

Cardiovascular Examination

- Heart: ....
- Heart sounds: ....
- Murmurs: ....
- Carotid pulse: ....
- Apical pulse: ....
- Peripheral pulses: ....
- Blood pressure: .... Pulse rate: ....

Abdominal Examination

- Contour: ....
- Skin: ....
- Bowel sounds: ....
- On percussion: ....
- Palpation: ....

Musculoskeletal Examination

- Back: ....
- Vertebral column alignment: ....
- Joints: ....
- Range of motion: ....
- Extremities: ....
- Lower extremities: ....

Genitourinary and Rectum Inspection

- Rectum: ....
- Female genitalia: ....
- Male genitalia: ....

Neurological Examination

- Describe tics, twitches, paresthesia: ....
- Gait: ....
- Accessory (CN XI): ....
- Reflex: ....
- Coordination: ....
- Cranial nerves: ....

Mental Status Examination

- Level of alertness: ....
- Orientation: ....
- Memory: ....
- Language and speech: ....
- Responsiveness: ....
- Knowledge test: ....
- Thinking: ....
- Judgment: ....
- Insight: ....

Final Impression and Suspected Illness/Disease (States the Problem or Nursing Diagnosis)

....

....

....

....

....

CASE 5

PHYSICAL EXAMINATION

Name of the Patient: .... **Age:** .... **Sex:** ....

Educational Status: ....

Date of Admission: .... **IP No:** .... **MLC/OP No:** ....

Medical Diagnosis: ....

General Appearance

- Level of consciousness: ....
- Activity: ....
- Body built: ....
- Height: ....
- Weight: ....
- Mid-upper arm circumference: ....
- General grooming: ....
- Position/Posturing: ....
- Facial expression: ....
- Body language: ....
- Other observations: ....

Skin Inspection and Palpation

- Color and vascularity: ....
- Turgor and mobility: ....
- Temperature and moisture: ....
- Texture: ....
- Nails: ....
- Body hair growth: ....
- Skin integrity: ....
- Lesions: ....

Head Inspection and Palpation

- Shape: ....
- Face: ....
- Sensations (CN V): ....

- Facial (CN V): ....
- Hair: ....
- Condition of scalp: ....
- Masses and lumps: ....
- Facial puffiness: ....

Eyes Inspection and Palpation

- Eyebrows: ....
- Eyelashes: ....
- Eyelids: ....
- Shape and appearance: ....
- Sclera: ....
- Conjunctiva: ....
- Iris: ....
- Cornea: ....
- Pupils: ....
- Visual field: ....
- Vision: ....
- Use of glasses: ....

Ears Inspection and Palpation

- Pinnae: ....
- Level in relation to eyes: ....
- Canal: ....
- Cilia: ....
- Cerumen: ....
- Tympanic membrane: ....
- Hearing (audition-CN VIII): ....
- Tuning fork test: ....
- Weber test: ....
- Rinne test: ....
- Hearing aid: ....

Nose and Sinuses Inspection and Palpation

- Size and shape: ....
- Nasal septum: ....

- Nasal mucosa and turbinate: ....
- Patency of nares: ....
- Olfactory (CN I): ....
- Sinuses: ....

Mouth and Pharynx Inspection

- Lips: ....
- Teeth: ....
- Dental caries and fillings: ....
- Dental hygiene: ....
- Breath odor: ....
- Gums: ....
- Facial and glossopharyngeal (CN VII and IX): ....
- Tongue: ....
- Hypoglossal (CN XII): ....
- Mucosa: ....
- Palate: ....
- Uvula: ....
- Pharynx: ....
- Tonsils: ....
- Temporomandibular joint: ....

Neck Inspection and Palpation

- Appearance: ....
- Thyroid: ....
- Trachea: ....
- Lymph nodes: ....

Thorax and Lung Examination

- Respiratory rate: ....
- Thoracic cage shape: ....
- Configuration: ....
- Skin color and condition: ....
- Chest examination: ....
- Posterior thorax: ....

- Percussion on lung field: ....
- Diaphragmatic exertion: ....
- Lung auscultation: ....
- Breath sound: ....
- Respiratory pattern: ....

Breasts and Axillae Inspection and Palpation

- Male breasts: ....
- Female breasts: ....
- Nipples: ....
- Axilla: ....

Cardiovascular Examination

- Heart: ....
- Heart sounds: ....
- Murmurs: ....
- Carotid pulse: ....
- Apical pulse: ....
- Peripheral pulses: ....
- Blood pressure: .... Pulse rate: ....

Abdominal Examination

- Contour: ....
- Skin: ....
- Bowel sounds: ....
- On percussion: ....
- Palpation: ....

Musculoskeletal Examination

- Back: ....
- Vertebral column alignment: ....
- Joints: ....
- Range of motion: ....
- Extremities: ....
- Lower extremities: ....

Genitourinary and Rectum Inspection

- Rectum: ....
- Female genitalia: ....
- Male genitalia: ....

Neurological Examination

- Describe tics, twitches, paresthesia: ....
- Gait: ....
- Accessory (CN XI): ....
- Reflex: ....
- Coordination: ....
- Cranial nerves: ....

Mental Status Examination

- Level of alertness: ....
- Orientation: ....
- Memory: ....
- Language and speech: ....
- Responsiveness: ....
- Knowledge test: ....
- Thinking: ....
- Judgment: ....
- Insight: ....

Final Impression and Suspected Illness/Disease (States the Problem or Nursing Diagnosis)

....

....

....

....

....

SECTION III

CASE 1

Case Study/Case Presentation

BIOGRAPHICAL DATA

Name of the Patient: ....

Name of the Father/Guardian/Husband: ....

Date of Birth: .... Age: .... Sex: ....

Marital Status: .... Education: ....

Occupation: .... Monthly Income: ....

Mother Tongue: .... Religion: .... Nationality: ....

Educational Status: ....

Date of Admission: .... IP No: .... MLC/OP No: ....

Address: ....

....

....

Medical Diagnosis: .... Doctor's Name: ....

Name of the Hospital: ....

Ward: .... Bed Number: ....

Date of Data Collection/Care Started: ....

Date of Care Ended: ....

History of Present Illness (Medical/Surgical)

(Mention the onset of illness, i.e. pain, headache, fever, change in bowel habits, etc. effects on ADLs, precipitating factors and relief measures initiated, etc.)

Past History of Illness

(Mention any previous history of childhood illness, adult illness, psychiatric illness, injuries, hospitalization, surgical diagnosis, measures, current medications, use of alcohol and drugs.)

Family History

(Mention the location, type of family, number of family members, educational status, occupation, income, health status and any significant problems related to health of the family and the patient.)

Personal History

[Mention the ability to ADLs, IADLs, life style pattern (sleep, exercise, nutrition, recreation, smoking, alcohol, drugs, etc.), hygiene, activities, exercises, rest, sleep, elimination pattern, education, occupational status and source of income in brief, and menstrual history if female.]

Present Chief Complaints of Patient

Physical Examination

Note: Normal or any abnormalities related to health to be mentioned, as per descriptive terms suggested in guidelines, i.e:

1. General appearance: ....
2. Vital signs:
   - Temperature: ....
   - Pulse: ....
   - Respiratory rate: ....
   - Blood pressure (BP): ....
3. Head: ....
4. Face: ....
5. Eyes: ....
6. Ears: ....
7. Nose and sinuses: ....
8. Throat: ....
9. Mouth and pharynx: ....
10. Neck: ....
11. Thorax: ....
    - Respiration: ....
    - Posterior thorax: ....
    - Lung auscultation: ....
    - Breast and axillae: ....

Cardiovascular

- Heart sound: ....
- Peripheral vascular: ....

Gastrointestinal System

- Contour: ....
- Skin: ....
- Bowel sounds: ....
- Percussion: ....
- Palpation: ....

Integumentary System

- Color: ....
- Texture: ....
- Turgor: ....
- Temperature: ....

Musculoskeletal System

- Back: ....
- Vertebral column: ....
- Joints: ....
- Range of motion (ROM): ....
- Upper extremities: ....
- Lower extremities: ....

Genitourinary and Rectum

- Rectum: ....
- Female genitalia: ....
- Male genitalia: ....

Reproductive System

- Menstruation: ....
- Pregnancies: ....
- Breasts: ....

Neurological Assessment

- Gait: ....
- Reflexes: ....
- Coordination: ....
- Cranial nerves: ....

Mental Status

- Level of consciousness: ....
- Orientation: ....
- Memory: ....
- Language and speech: ....

List the Problems/Needs of the Patient

Actual Problems

1.
2.
3.
4.
5.

Potential Problems

1.
2.
3.
4.
5.

DESCRIPTION OF PRESENT DISEASE

Introduction

Definition

Related Anatomy and Physiology (brief note of organ involved with relevant diagram)

Etiology/Risk Factors (mention present causes, possible causes and risk factors, and can be compared with text)

Pathophysiology (mention the present pathophysiology of the patient and pathophysiology of particular disease explained in the text)

Clinical Manifestations

(List the sign and symptoms present in the patient, probable complications and same are explained in the text and compare.)

List Signs and Symptoms	Explained in the Text

Diagnostic Tests

Mention the indicated tests and performed tests:

- Laboratory test: ....
- Radiological test: ....
- Other tests: ....

Medical Management

(Mention the measures taken by the concerned doctors and team in brief.)

Medication	Dosage	Route	Frequency	Side Effects	Nurses Responsibility

Nursing Management

(List the nursing diagnosis or problems according to nursing assessment, draw a nursing care plan on priority, set objectives. Perform nursing interventions and evaluate accordingly.)

Nursing Diagnosis

1.
2.
3.
4.
5.

Objectives: To be shown in nursing care plan (NCP)

Interventions: To be shown in NCP

Nursing Care Plan

There are number of formats of nursing care plan used by different institutions, those can be used accordingly. Here some illustrations given below. Select anyone case from Section IV 'Nursing Care Plans'.

Note: Students are instructed to use separate sheets included in the application of nursing process.

Format 1:

Nursing Assessment	Nursing Diagnosis	Expected Outcome	Nursing Interventions	Rationale	Evaluation
Subjective data: .... Objective data:					

Format 2: PRONE

Problem	Reason	Objectives	Nursing Interventions	Evaluation
	Subjective data: .... Objective data:			

NURSES NOTES

Name of the Patient: .... Age: .... Sex: ....

Ward No: .... Bed No: .... Diagnosis: ....

Treatment: .... Name of Surgery (if any): ....

Date of Surgery: ....

Date	Medication	Diet	Time	Observation	Signature

Summary and Conclusion

Bibliography

1. Example: Basavanthappa BT. 'Medical Surgical Nursing' 3rd edition. Jaypee Brothers Medical Publishers (P) Ltd, New Delhi. 2014.
2.
3.

CASE 2

Case Study/Case Presentation

BIOGRAPHICAL DATA

Name of the Patient: ....

Name of the Father/Guardian/Husband: ....

Date of Birth: .... Age: .... Sex: ....

Marital Status: .... Education: ....

Occupation: .... Monthly Income: ....

Mother Tongue: .... Religion: .... Nationality: ....

Educational Status: ....

Date of Admission: .... IP No: .... MLC/OP No: ....

Address: ....

....

....

Medical Diagnosis: .... Doctor's Name: ....

Name of the Hospital: ....

Ward: .... Bed Number: ....

Date of Data Collection/Care Started: ....

Date of Care Ended: ....

History of Present Illness (Medical/Surgical)

(Mention the onset of illness, i.e. pain, headache, fever, change in bowel habits, etc. effects on ADLs, precipitating factors and relief measures initiated, etc.)

Past History of Illness

(Mention any previous history of childhood illness, adult illness, psychiatric illness, injuries, hospitalization, surgical diagnosis, measures, current medications, use of alcohol and drugs.)

Family History

(Mention the location, type of family, number of family members, educational status, occupation, income, health status and any significant problems related to health of the family and the patient.)

Personal History

[Mention the ability to ADLs, IADLs, life style pattern (sleep, exercise, nutrition, recreation, smoking, alcohol, drugs, etc.), hygiene, activities, exercises, rest, sleep, elimination pattern, education, occupational status and source of income in brief, and menstrual history if female.]

Present Chief Complaints of Patient

Physical Examination

Note: Normal or any abnormalities related to health to be mentioned, as per descriptive terms suggested in guidelines, i.e:

1. General appearance: ....
2. Vital signs:
   - Temperature: ....
   - Pulse: ....
   - Respiratory rate: ....
   - Blood pressure (BP): ....
3. Head: ....
4. Face: ....
5. Eyes: ....
6. Ears: ....
7. Nose and sinuses: ....
8. Throat: ....
9. Mouth and pharynx: ....
10. Neck: ....
11. Thorax: ....
    - Respiration: ....
    - Posterior thorax: ....
    - Lung auscultation: ....
    - Breast and axillae: ....

Cardiovascular

- Heart sound: ....
- Peripheral vascular: ....

Gastrointestinal System

- Contour: ....
- Skin: ....
- Bowel sounds: ....
- Percussion: ....
- Palpation: ....

Integumentary System

- Color: ....
- Texture: ....
- Turgor: ....
- Temperature: ....

Musculoskeletal System

- Back: ....
- Vertebral column: ....
- Joints: ....
- Range of motion (ROM): ....
- Upper extremities: ....
- Lower extremities: ....

Genitourinary and Rectum

- Rectum: ....
- Female genitalia: ....
- Male genitalia: ....

Reproductive System

- Menstruation: ....
- Pregnancies: ....
- Breasts: ....

Neurological Assessment

- Gait: ....
- Reflexes: ....
- Coordination: ....
- Cranial nerves: ....

Mental Status

- Level of consciousness: ....
- Orientation: ....
- Memory: ....
- Language and speech: ....

List the Problems/Needs of the Patient

Actual Problems

1.
2.
3.
4.
5.

Potential Problems

1.
2.
3.
4.
5.

DESCRIPTION OF PRESENT DISEASE

Introduction

Definition

Related Anatomy and Physiology (brief note of organ involved with relevant diagram)

Etiology/Risk Factors (mention present causes, possible causes and risk factors, and can be compared with text)

Pathophysiology (mention the present pathophysiology of the patient and pathophysiology of particular disease explained in the text)

Clinical Manifestations

(List the sign and symptoms present in the patient, probable complications and same are explained in the text and compare.)

List Signs and Symptoms	Explained in the Text

Diagnostic Tests

Mention the indicated tests and performed tests:

- Laboratory test: ....
- Radiological test: ....
- Other tests: ....

Medical Management

(Mention the measures taken by the concerned doctors and team in brief.)

Medication	Dosage	Route	Frequency	Side Effects	Nurses Responsibility

Nursing Management

(List the nursing diagnosis or problems according to nursing assessment, draw a nursing care plan on priority, set objectives. Perform nursing interventions and evaluate accordingly.)

Nursing Diagnosis

1.
2.
3.
4.
5.

Objectives: To be shown in nursing care plan (NCP)

Interventions: To be shown in NCP

Nursing Care Plan

There are number of formats of nursing care plan used by different institutions, those can be used accordingly. Here some illustrations given below. Select anyone case from Section IV 'Nursing Care Plans.'

Note: Students are instructed to use separate sheets included in the application of nursing process.

Format 1:

Nursing Assessment	Nursing Diagnosis	Expected Outcome	Nursing Interventions	Rationale	Evaluation
Subjective data: .... Objective data:					

Format 2: PRONE

Problem	Reason	Objectives	Nursing Interventions	Evaluation
	Subjective data: .... Objective data:			

NURSES NOTES

Name of the Patient: .... Age: .... Sex: ....

Ward No: .... Bed No: .... Diagnosis: ....

Treatment: .... Name of Surgery (if any): ....

Date of Surgery: ....

Date	Medication	Diet	Time	Observation	Signature

Summary and Conclusion

Bibliography

1. Example: Basavanthappa BT. 'Medical Surgical Nursing' 3rd edition. Jaypee Brothers Medical Publishers (P) Ltd, New Delhi. 2014.
2.
3.

CASE 3

Case Study/Case Presentation

BIOGRAPHICAL DATA

Name of the Patient: ....

Name of the Father/Guardian/Husband: ....

Date of Birth: .... Age: .... Sex: ....

Marital Status: .... Education: ....

Occupation: .... Monthly Income: ....

Mother Tongue: .... Religion: .... Nationality: ....

Educational Status: ....

Date of Admission: .... IP No: .... MLC/OP No: ....

Address: ....

....

....

Medical Diagnosis: .... Doctor's Name: ....

Name of the Hospital: ....

Ward: .... Bed Number: ....

Date of Data Collection/Care Started: ....

Date of Care Ended: ....

History of Present Illness (Medical/Surgical)

(Mention the onset of illness, i.e. pain, headache, fever, change in bowel habits, etc. effects on ADLs, precipitating factors and relief measures initiated, etc.)

Past History of Illness

(Mention any previous history of childhood illness, adult illness, psychiatric illness, injuries, hospitalization, surgical diagnosis, measures, current medications, use of alcohol and drugs.)

Family History

(Mention the location, type of family, number of family members, educational status, occupation, income, health status and any significant problems related to health of the family and the patient.)

Personal History

[Mention the ability to ADLs, IADLs, life style pattern (sleep, exercise, nutrition, recreation, smoking, alcohol, drugs, etc.), hygiene, activities, exercises, rest, sleep, elimination pattern, education, occupational status and source of income in brief, and menstrual history if female.]

Present Chief Complaints of Patient

Physical Examination

Note: Normal or any abnormalities related to health to be mentioned, as per descriptive terms suggested in guidelines, i.e:

1. General appearance: ....
2. Vital signs:
    - Temperature: ....
    - Pulse: ....
    - Respiratory rate: ....
    - Blood pressure (BP): ....
3. Head: ....
4. Face: ....
5. Eyes: ....
6. Ears: ....
7. Nose and sinuses: ....
8. Throat: ....
9. Mouth and pharynx: ....
10. Neck: ....
11. Thorax: ....
    - Respiration: ....
    - Posterior thorax: ....
    - Lung auscultation: ....
    - Breast and axillae: ....

Cardiovascular

- Heart sound: ....
- Peripheral vascular: ....

Gastrointestinal System

- Contour: ....
- Skin: ....
- Bowel sounds: ....
- Percussion: ....
- Palpation: ....

Integumentary System

- Color: ....
- Texture: ....
- Turgor: ....
- Temperature: ....

Musculoskeletal System

- Back: ....
- Vertebral column: ....
- Joints: ....
- Range of motion (ROM): ....
- Upper extremities: ....
- Lower extremities: ....

Genitourinary and Rectum

- Rectum: ....
- Female genitalia: ....
- Male genitalia: ....

Reproductive System

- Menstruation: ....
- Pregnancies: ....
- Breasts: ....

Neurological Assessment

- Gait: ....
- Reflexes: ....
- Coordination: ....
- Cranial nerves: ....

Mental Status

- Level of consciousness: ....
- Orientation: ....
- Memory: ....
- Language and speech: ....

List the Problems/Needs of the Patient

Actual Problems

1.
2.
3.
4.
5.

Potential Problems

1.
2.
3.
4.
5.

DESCRIPTION OF PRESENT DISEASE

Introduction

Definition

Related Anatomy and Physiology (brief note of organ involved with relevant diagram)

Etiology/Risk Factors (mention present causes, possible causes and risk factors, and can be compared with text)

Pathophysiology (mention the present pathophysiology of the patient and pathophysiology of particular disease explained in the text)

Clinical Manifestations

(List the sign and symptoms present in the patient, probable complications and same are explained in the text and compare.)

List Signs and Symptoms	Explained in the Text

Diagnostic Tests

Mention the indicated tests and performed tests:

- Laboratory test: ....
- Radiological test: ....
- Other tests: ....

Medical Management

(Mention the measures taken by the concerned doctors and team in brief.)

Medication	Dosage	Route	Frequency	Side Effects	Nurses Responsibility

Nursing Management

(List the nursing diagnosis or problems according to nursing assessment, draw a nursing care plan on priority, set objectives. Perform nursing interventions and evaluate accordingly.)

Nursing Diagnosis

1.
2.
3.
4.
5.

Objectives: To be shown in nursing care plan (NCP)

Interventions: To be shown in NCP

Nursing Care Plan

There are number of formats of nursing care plan used by different institutions, those can be used accordingly. Here some illustrations given below. Select anyone case from Section IV 'Nursing Care Plans.'

Note: Students are instructed to use separate sheets included in the application of nursing process.

Format 1:

Nursing Assessment	Nursing Diagnosis	Expected Outcome	Nursing Interventions	Rationale	Evaluation
Subjective data: .... Objective data:					

Format 2: PRONE

Problem	Reason	Objectives	Nursing Interventions	Evaluation
	Subjective data: .... Objective data:			

NURSES NOTES

Name of the Patient: .... Age: .... Sex: ....

Ward No: .... Bed No: .... Diagnosis: ....

Treatment: .... Name of Surgery (if any): ....

Date of Surgery: ....

Date	Medication	Diet	Time	Observation	Signature

Summary and Conclusion

Bibliography

1. Example: Basavanthappa BT. 'Medical Surgical Nursing' 3rd edition. Jaypee Brothers Medical Publishers (P) Ltd, New Delhi. 2014.
2.
3.

CASE 4

Case Study/Case Presentation

BIOGRAPHICAL DATA

Name of the Patient: ....

Name of the Father/Guardian/Husband: ....

Date of Birth: .... Age: .... Sex: ....

Marital Status: .... Education: ....

Occupation: .... Monthly Income: ....

Mother Tongue: .... Religion: .... Nationality: ....

Educational Status: ....

Date of Admission: .... IP No: .... MLC/OP No: ....

Address: ....

....

....

Medical Diagnosis: .... Doctor's Name: ....

Name of the Hospital: ....

Ward: .... Bed Number: ....

Date of Data Collection/Care Started: ....

Date of Care Ended: ....

History of Present Illness (Medical/Surgical)

(Mention the onset of illness, i.e. pain, headache, fever, change in bowel habits, etc. effects on ADLs, precipitating factors and relief measures initiated, etc.)

Past History of Illness

(Mention any previous history of childhood illness, adult illness, psychiatric illness, injuries, hospitalization, surgical diagnosis, measures, current medications, use of alcohol and drugs.)

Family History

(Mention the location, type of family, number of family members, educational status, occupation, income, health status and any significant problems related to health of the family and the patient.)

Personal History

[Mention the ability to ADLs, IADLs, life style pattern (sleep, exercise, nutrition, recreation, smoking, alcohol, drugs, etc.), hygiene, activities, exercises, rest, sleep, elimination pattern, education, occupational status and source of income in brief, and menstrual history if female.]

Present Chief Complaints of Patient

Physical Examination

Note: Normal or any abnormalities related to health to be mentioned, as per descriptive terms suggested in guidelines, i.e:

1. General appearance: ....
2. Vital signs:
   - Temperature: ....
   - Pulse: ....
   - Respiratory rate: ....
   - Blood pressure (BP): ....
3. Head: ....
4. Face: ....
5. Eyes: ....
6. Ears: ....
7. Nose and sinuses: ....
8. Throat: ....
9. Mouth and pharynx: ....
10. Neck: ....
11. Thorax: ....
    - Respiration: ....
    - Posterior thorax: ....
    - Lung auscultation: ....
    - Breast and axillae: ....

Cardiovascular

- Heart sound: ....
- Peripheral vascular: ....

Gastrointestinal System

- Contour: ....
- Skin: ....
- Bowel sounds: ....
- Percussion: ....
- Palpation: ....

Integumentary System

- Color: ....
- Texture: ....
- Turgor: ....
- Temperature: ....

Musculoskeletal System

- Back: ....
- Vertebral column: ....
- Joints: ....
- Range of motion (ROM): ....
- Upper extremities: ....
- Lower extremities: ....

Genitourinary and Rectum

- Rectum: ....
- Female genitalia: ....
- Male genitalia: ....

Reproductive System

- Menstruation: ....
- Pregnancies: ....
- Breasts: ....

Neurological Assessment

- Gait: ....
- Reflexes: ....
- Coordination: ....
- Cranial nerves: ....

Mental Status

- Level of consciousness: ....
- Orientation: ....
- Memory: ....
- Language and speech: ....

List the Problems/Needs of the Patient

Actual Problems

1.
2.
3.
4.
5.

Potential Problems

1.
2.
3.
4.
5.

DESCRIPTION OF PRESENT DISEASE

Introduction

Definition

Related Anatomy and Physiology (brief note of organ involved with relevant diagram)

Etiology/Risk Factors (mention present causes, possible causes and risk factors, and can be compared with text)

Pathophysiology (mention the present pathophysiology of the patient and pathophysiology of particular disease explained in the text)

Clinical Manifestations

(List the sign and symptoms present in the patient, probable complications and same are explained in the text and compare.)

List Signs and Symptoms	Explained in the Text

Diagnostic Tests

Mention the indicated tests and performed tests:

- Laboratory test: ....
- Radiological test: ....
- Other tests: ....

Medical Management

(Mention the measures taken by the concerned doctors and team in brief.)

Medication	Dosage	Route	Frequency	Side Effects	Nurses Responsibility

Nursing Management

(List the nursing diagnosis or problems according to nursing assessment, draw a nursing care plan on priority, set objectives. Perform nursing interventions and evaluate accordingly.)

Nursing Diagnosis

1.
2.
3.
4.
5.

Objectives: To be shown in nursing care plan (NCP)

Interventions: To be shown in NCP

Nursing Care Plan

There are number of formats of nursing care plan used by different institutions, those can be used accordingly. Here some illustrations given below. Select anyone case from Section IV 'Nursing Care Plans'.

Note: Students are instructed to use separate sheets included in the application of nursing process.

Format 1:

Nursing Assessment	Nursing Diagnosis	Expected Outcome	Nursing Interventions	Rationale	Evaluation
Subjective data: .... Objective data:					

Format 2: PRONE

Problem	Reason	Objectives	Nursing Interventions	Evaluation
	Subjective data: .... Objective data:			

NURSES NOTES

Name of the Patient: .... Age: .... Sex: ....

Ward No: .... Bed No: .... Diagnosis: ....

Treatment: .... Name of Surgery (if any): ....

Date of Surgery: ....

Date	Medication	Diet	Time	Observation	Signature

Summary and Conclusion

Bibliography

1. Example: Basavanthappa BT. 'Medical Surgical Nursing' 3rd edition. Jaypee Brothers Medical Publishers (P) Ltd, New Delhi. 2014.
2.
3.

CASE 5

Case Study/Case Presentation

BIOGRAPHICAL DATA

Name of the Patient: ....

Name of the Father/Guardian/Husband: ....

Date of Birth: .... Age: .... Sex: ....

Marital Status: .... Education: ....

Occupation: .... Monthly Income: ....

Mother Tongue: .... Religion: .... Nationality: ....

Educational Status: ....

Date of Admission: .... IP No: .... MLC/OP No: ....

Address: ....

....

....

Medical Diagnosis: .... Doctor's Name: ....

Name of the Hospital: ....

Ward: .... Bed Number: ....

Date of Data Collection/Care Started: ....

Date of Care Ended: ....

History of Present Illness (Medical/Surgical)

(Mention the onset of illness, i.e. pain, headache, fever, change in bowel habits, etc. effects on ADLs, precipitating factors and relief measures initiated, etc.)

Past History of Illness

(Mention any previous history of childhood illness, adult illness, psychiatric illness, injuries, hospitalization, surgical diagnosis, measures, current medications, use of alcohol and drugs.)

Family History

(Mention the location, type of family, number of family members, educational status, occupation, income, health status and any significant problems related to health of the family and the patient.)

Personal History

[Mention the ability to ADLs, IADLs, life style pattern (sleep, exercise, nutrition, recreation, smoking, alcohol, drugs, etc.), hygiene, activities, exercises, rest, sleep, elimination pattern, education, occupational status and source of income in brief, and menstrual history if female.]

Present Chief Complaints of Patient

Physical Examination

Note: Normal or any abnormalities related to health to be mentioned, as per descriptive terms suggested in guidelines, i.e:

1. General appearance: ....
2. Vital signs:
   - Temperature: ....
   - Pulse: ....
   - Respiratory rate: ....
   - Blood pressure (BP): ....
3. Head: ....
4. Face: ....
5. Eyes: ....
6. Ears: ....
7. Nose and sinuses: ....
8. Throat: ....
9. Mouth and pharynx: ....
10. Neck: ....
11. Thorax: ....
    - Respiration: ....
    - Posterior thorax: ....
    - Lung auscultation: ....
    - Breast and axillae: ....

Cardiovascular

- Heart sound: ....
- Peripheral vascular: ....

Gastrointestinal System

- Contour: ....
- Skin: ....
- Bowel sounds: ....
- Percussion: ....
- Palpation: ....

Integumentary System

- Color: ....
- Texture: ....
- Turgor: ....
- Temperature: ....

Musculoskeletal System

- Back: ....
- Vertebral column: ....
- Joints: ....
- Range of motion (ROM): ....
- Upper extremities: ....
- Lower extremities: ....

Genitourinary and Rectum

- Rectum: ....
- Female genitalia: ....
- Male genitalia: ....

Reproductive System

- Menstruation: ....
- Pregnancies: ....
- Breasts: ....

Neurological Assessment

- Gait:...
- Reflexes:...
- Coordination: ....
- Cranial nerves: ....

Mental Status

- Level of consciousness: ....
- Orientation: ....
- Memory: ....
- Language and speech: ....

List the Problems/Needs of the Patient

Actual Problems

1.
2.
3.
4.
5.

Potential Problems

1.
2.
3.
4.
5.

DESCRIPTION OF PRESENT DISEASE

Introduction

Definition

Related Anatomy and Physiology (brief note of organ involved with relevant diagram)

Etiology/Risk Factors (mention present causes, possible causes and risk factors, and can be compared with text)

Pathophysiology (mention the present pathophysiology of the patient and pathophysiology of particular disease explained in the text)

Clinical Manifestations

(List the sign and symptoms present in the patient, probable complications and same are explained in the text and compare.)

List Signs and Symptoms	Explained in the Text

Diagnostic Tests

Mention the indicated tests and performed tests:

- Laboratory test: ....
- Radiological test: ....
- Other tests: ....

Medical Management

(Mention the measures taken by the concerned doctors and team in brief.)

Medication	Dosage	Route	Frequency	Side Effects	Nurses Responsibility

Nursing Management

(List the nursing diagnosis or problems according to nursing assessment, draw a nursing care plan on priority, set objectives. Perform nursing interventions and evaluate accordingly.)

Nursing Diagnosis

1.
2.
3.
4.
5.

Objectives: To be shown in nursing care plan (NCP)

Interventions: To be shown in NCP

Nursing Care Plan

There are number of formats of nursing care plan used by different institutions, those can be used accordingly. Here some illustrations given below. Select anyone case from Section IV 'Nursing Care Plans.'

Note: Students are instructed to use separate sheets included in the application of nursing process.

Format 1:

Nursing Assessment	Nursing Diagnosis	Expected Outcome	Nursing Interventions	Rationale	Evaluation
Subjective data: .... Objective data:					

Format 2: PRONE

Problem	Reason	Objectives	Nursing Interventions	Evaluation
	Subjective data: .... Objective data:			

NURSES NOTES

Name of the Patient: .... Age: .... Sex: ....

Ward No: .... Bed No: .... Diagnosis: ....

Treatment: .... Name of Surgery (if any): ....

Date of Surgery: ....

Date	Medication	Diet	Time	Observation	Signature

Summary and Conclusion

Bibliography

1. Example: Basavanthappa BT. 'Medical Surgical Nursing' 3rd edition. Jaypee Brothers Medical Publishers (P) Ltd, New Delhi. 2014.
2.
3.

CASE 6

Case Study/Case Presentation

BIOGRAPHICAL DATA

Name of the Patient: ....

Name of the Father/Guardian/Husband: ....

Date of Birth: .... Age: .... Sex: ....

Marital Status: .... Education: ....

Occupation: .... Monthly Income: ....

Mother Tongue: .... Religion: .... Nationality: ....

Educational Status: ....

Date of Admission: .... IP No: .... MLC/OP No: ....

Address: ....

....

....

Medical Diagnosis: .... Doctor's Name: ....

Name of the Hospital: ....

Ward: .... Bed Number: ....

Date of Data Collection/Care Started: ....

Date of Care Ended: ....

History of Present Illness (Medical/Surgical)

(Mention the onset of illness, i.e. pain, headache, fever, change in bowel habits, etc. effects on ADLs, precipitating factors and relief measures initiated, etc.)

Past History of Illness

(Mention any previous history of childhood illness, adult illness, psychiatric illness, injuries, hospitalization, surgical diagnosis, measures, current medications, use of alcohol and drugs.)

Family History

(Mention the location, type of family, number of family members, educational status, occupation, income, health status and any significant problems related to health of the family and the patient.)

Personal History

[Mention the ability to ADLs, IADLs, life style pattern (sleep, exercise, nutrition, recreation, smoking, alcohol, drugs, etc.), hygiene, activities, exercises, rest, sleep, elimination pattern, education, occupational status and source of income in brief, and menstrual history if female.]

Present Chief Complaints of Patient

Physical Examination

Note: Normal or any abnormalities related to health to be mentioned, as per descriptive terms suggested in guidelines, i.e:

1. General appearance: ....
2. Vital signs:
   - Temperature: ....
   - Pulse: ....
   - Respiratory rate: ....
   - Blood pressure (BP): ....
3. Head: ....
4. Face: ....
5. Eyes: ....
6. Ears: ....
7. Nose and sinuses: ....
8. Throat: ....
9. Mouth and pharynx: ....
10. Neck: ....
11. Thorax: ....
    - Respiration: ....
    - Posterior thorax: ....
    - Lung auscultation: ....
    - Breast and axillae: ....

Cardiovascular

- Heart sound: ....
- Peripheral vascular: ....

Gastrointestinal System

- Contour: ....
- Skin: ....
- Bowel sounds: ....
- Percussion: ....
- Palpation: ....

Integumentary System

- Color: ....
- Texture: ....
- Turgor: ....
- Temperature: ....

Musculoskeletal System

- Back: ....
- Vertebral column: ....
- Joints: ....
- Range of motion (ROM): ....
- Upper extremities: ....
- Lower extremities: ....

Genitourinary and Rectum

- Rectum: ....
- Female genitalia: ....
- Male genitalia: ....

Reproductive System

- Menstruation: ....
- Pregnancies: ....
- Breasts: ....

Neurological Assessment

- Gait: ....
- Reflexes: ....
- Coordination: ....
- Cranial nerves: ....

Mental Status

- Level of consciousness: ....
- Orientation: ....
- Memory: ....
- Language and speech: ....

List the Problems/Needs of the Patient

Actual Problems

1.
2.
3.
4.
5.

Potential Problems

1.
2.
3.
4.
5.

DESCRIPTION OF PRESENT DISEASE

Introduction

Definition

Related Anatomy and Physiology (brief note of organ involved with relevant diagram)

Etiology/Risk Factors (mention present causes, possible causes and risk factors, and can be compared with text)

Pathophysiology (mention the present pathophysiology of the patient and pathophysiology of particular disease explained in the text)

Clinical Manifestations

(List the sign and symptoms present in the patient, probable complications and same are explained in the text and compare.)

List Signs and Symptoms	Explained in the Text

Diagnostic Tests

Mention the indicated tests and performed tests:

- Laboratory test: ....
- Radiological test: ....
- Other tests: ....

Medical Management

(Mention the measures taken by the concerned doctors and team in brief.)

Medication	Dosage	Route	Frequency	Side Effects	Nurses Responsibility

Nursing Management

(List the nursing diagnosis or problems according to nursing assessment, draw a nursing care plan on priority, set objectives. Perform nursing interventions and evaluate accordingly.)

Nursing Diagnosis

1.
2.
3.
4.
5.

Objectives: To be shown in nursing care plan (NCP)

Interventions: To be shown in NCP

Nursing Care Plan

There are number of formats of nursing care plan used by different institutions, those can be used accordingly. Here some illustrations given below. Select anyone case from Section IV 'Nursing Care Plans.'

Note: Students are instructed to use separate sheets included in the application of nursing process.

Format 1:

Nursing Assessment	Nursing Diagnosis	Expected Outcome	Nursing Interventions	Rationale	Evaluation
Subjective data: .... Objective data:					

Format 2: PRONE

Problem	Reason	Objectives	Nursing Interventions	Evaluation
	Subjective data: .... Objective data:			

NURSES NOTES

Name of the Patient: .... Age: .... Sex: ....

Ward No: .... Bed No: .... Diagnosis: ....

Treatment: .... Name of Surgery (if any): ....

Date of Surgery: ....

Date	Medication	Diet	Time	Observation	Signature

Summary and Conclusion

Bibliography

1. Example: Basavanthappa BT. 'Medical Surgical Nursing' 3rd edition. Jaypee Brothers Medical Publishers (P) Ltd, New Delhi. 2014.
2.
3.

SECTION IV

NURSING CARE PLAN

Guidelines for Application of Nursing Process

REVIEW OF NURSING PROCESS

Nursing is the diagnosis and treatment of human responses to actual or potential problems. The fundamental basis of nursing practice is known as 'process'. Process is the series of actions or steps toward achieving a particular end. Nursing process is an organized approach to problem solving and decision making that describes the intellectual activity of the nurse. The nursing process is the underlying source that provides order and direction of nursing care.

Meaning

- The nursing process is a deliberate intellectual activity by which the practice of nursing is approached in an orderly and systematic manner
- The nursing process is a systematic rational method of planning and providing individualized nursing care for individuals, families, group and communities.

Goals

The goal of nursing process are to identify a client's actual or potential healthcare needs, to establish plan to meet the identified needs, and to deliver and evaluate specific nursing interventions to meet those needs.

Steps

The nursing process can be used in all healthcare settings. It is cyclic and dynamic, client-centered, interpersonal and collaborative, universally applicable and focuses on problem solving and decision making. It is organized into five interrelated independent phases, i.e. assessing, diagnosing, planning, implementing and evaluating.

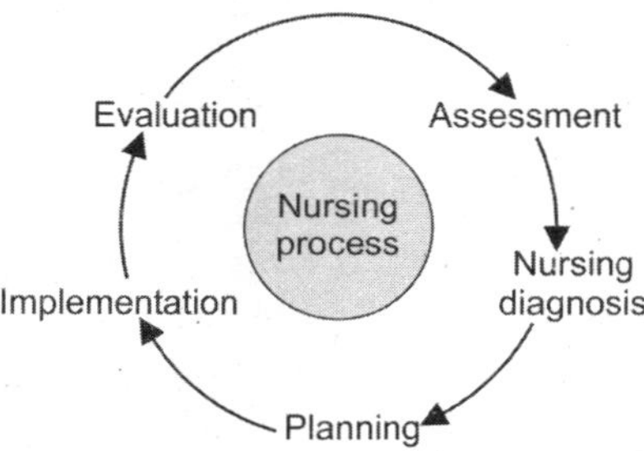

Assessment

Assessment involves collecting, organizing, validating and recording the data. It involves active participation by the client and nurse in obtaining subjective and objective data about the client's health status. Subjective data are the client's personal perception, often gathered during the nursing health history. Objective data are observed and collected during the physical examination, and are detectable by an observer.

Subjective data are symptoms that are documented in client's own words such as previous experiences, sensation and emotional as described or complained by the client.

Objective data are signs of clients obtained by the nurse or health team members through observation, physical examination or diagnostic tests that can be seen and measured.

Diagnosis

Diagnosis is the process of making a clinical judgment, i.e. nursing diagnosis about client's potential or actual health problem. Nursing diagnosis provides the basis for independent nursing intervention to achieve outcome for which nurse is accountable. Diagnostic process involves data analysis, identification of client health problems, health risks and strengths, and formulation of diagnostic statements, i.e. problem related to etiology.

Planning

Planning involves setting of priorities writing goals/objectives/desired outcomes and establishing a writing plan for nursing interventions (e.g. 'Nursing Care Plan' as shown in Section IV). It is process of designing nursing activities required to prevent, reduce or eliminate a client's health problems. Goals statement and desired outcomes or objectives are written in terms of client's behavior. Nursing interventions and activities are focused on the etiology of the nursing diagnosis.

Implementation

Implementation is carrying out the nursing interventions. It incorporates all the activities performed to promote health, prevent complications, treat present problem and facilitate the client to cope with chronic alterations in health status. The process of implementing involves reassessing the client, determining the nurses need for assistance, implementing the nursing interventions, supervision of the delegated care and documenting nursing activities. Here nurses actions include monitor the patient condition, perform direct patient care, educate the patient or caregivers and manage or refer to patient for further care or contact. Type of interventions may be independent, dependent or collaborative.

Evaluation

Evaluation is the process of comparing client's responses to preselected outcomes and to determine whether goals or objectives have been met. It includes review and modification of the care plan. Each nursing diagnosis or problem requires an actual outcome depicting of the outcome of care resulting from the intervention and action types used to treat or care of the patient. The same terms are used to predict the expected outcomes or care goals to evaluate whether the goals or objectives were met or not. The nursing diagnosis, collaborative problems, priorities, nursing interventions and expected outcomes provide the specific guidelines that dictate the focus of evaluation .The activities included in the evaluations are:

- Collect data about client's response
- Compare the client's response to goals and outcomes criteria/objectives
- The goal was completely met/partially met/completely unmet and more problems arised, e.g. to relive pain is the objective, it can be stated in evaluation as pain relieved, etc.
- Analyze the reasons for the outcomes
- Modify the plan and care as needed.

Nursing Care Plan (PRONE Format)

The nursing care plan (NCP) format is used throughout this text to afford the students the opportunity to examine the interrelatedness of the components of the nursing process, which includes problem, reason, objectives, nursing intervention (with rationale) and evaluation (PRONE) format.

Problem refers to the actual or potential problems, stated in the form of nursing diagnosis, which is the product of assessment.

Reason refers to an inference in the diagnostic reasoning. Diagnostic reasoning is the critical thinking process through which the nurse moves to arrive at a nursing diagnosis, which includes the key point of subjective data (client complaints) and objective data.

Objectives refer to short statement of desired or expected outcomes of the patient, in the subphase of planning component of nursing process.

Nursing intervention refers planned interventions, which will provide clarity, specificity and direction to the spectrum of nurses implementing care for a patient. Implementation of nursing intervention is the action component of the planning. It is the phase of the nursing process in which the nursing treatment plan is carried out.

Evaluation of the attainment of the expected patient outcome occurs formally at intervals designated in the outcome criteria. Please note that evaluation column is not included in the nursing care plans presented in this text, because they need to be individualized for each patient.

Author used the following 'PRONE' format for nursing care plan where 'P' stands for problem, 'R' stands for reason and 'O' stands for objectives. This is where and 'N' stands for nursing intervention and 'E' stands for evaluation. The sample of nursing care plan 'PRONE' format is as shown below (both are same as shown below).

Nursing Care Plan (PRONE Format)

Problem	Reason	Objective	Nursing Interventions with or Without Rationale	Evaluation

Nursing Care Plan—Other Format

Nursing Assessment (Reason)	Nursing of Diagnosis (Problem)	Expected Outcome (Objectives)	Nursing Interventions	Evaluation

Sample of Nursing Care Plan (PRONE Format)

Name: Revanna

Age: 50 years

Medical diagnosis: Benign prostate hypertrophy

	Problem	Reason	Objective	Nursing Interventions With or Without Rationale	Evaluation
1.	Anxiety related to unfamiliar disease condition	Patient express fear about hospital for surgery On observation: • Patient looks worried • Restlessness • Elevated BP • Looks pallor • Tachycardia	Relieve anxiety	• Assess the patient for signs and symptoms of fear, and anxiety like change in facial expressions, elevated blood pressure (BP), tachycardia, etc. • Place the patient in comfortable bed • Implement measures to reduce anxiety • Encourage verbalization of fear and provide feedback • Establish good rapport with the patient • Orient to hospital environment, equipment and routine • Be a good listener and adviser • Explain about the diagnostic tests to gain cooperation – Explain about the need for surgery – Possible result for surgery • Reassure the patient • Encourage the pertinent participating in diverse activities	Anxiety is relieved

Note: Students are advice to use any format for Nursing Care Plan on according their option or as instructed by your supervisor or HOD.

List of Nursing Care Plan made during Clinicals

Sl No	Patient Name	Age	Sex	Diagnosis

NURSING CARE PLAN NO. 1

Note 1: Students are advised to write at least 10 points on nursing care plan for selected case study and case presentation.

Note 2: Students are advised to write nursing care plan for the patient' problem or nursing diagnosis on priority basis with at least 5–6 identified actual or potential problems, and can also state accordingly short- or long-term goals and intervention accordingly.

Name of the Patient: ....

Age: ....

Sex: ....

Diagnosis: ....

Date of Care Started:

Nursing Assessment (Reason)	Nursing Diagnosis (Problem)	Expected Outcome (Objective)	Nursing Interventions	Rationale	Evaluation
Subjective data: .... Objective data:					

Contd...

Contd...

Nursing Assessment (Reason)	Nursing Diagnosis (Problem)	Expected Outcome (Objective)	Nursing Interventions	Rationale	Evaluation
Subjective data: .... Objective data:					

NURSING CARE PLAN NO. 2

Note 1: Students are advised to write at least 10 points on nursing care plan for selected case study and case presentation.

Note 2: Students are advised to write nursing care plan for the patient' problem or nursing diagnosis on priority basis with at least 5–6 identified actual or potential problems, and can also state accordingly short- or long-term goals and intervention accordingly.

Name of the Patient: ....

Age: ....

Sex: ....

Diagnosis: ....

Date of Care Started:

Nursing Assessment (Reason)	Nursing Diagnosis (Problem)	Expected Outcome (Objective)	Nursing Interventions	Rationale	Evaluation
Subjective data: .... Objective data:					

Contd...

Contd...

Nursing Assessment (Reason)	Nursing Diagnosis (Problem)	Expected Outcome (Objective)	Nursing Interventions	Rationale	Evaluation
Subjective data: .... Objective data:					

NURSING CARE PLAN NO. 3

Note 1: Students are advised to write at least 10 points on nursing care plan for selected case study and case presentation.

Note 2: Students are advised to write nursing care plan for the patient' problem or nursing diagnosis on priority basis with at least 5–6 identified actual or potential problems, and can also state accordingly short- or long-term goals and intervention accordingly.

Name of the Patient: ....

Age: ....

Sex: ....

Diagnosis: ....

Date of Care Started:

Nursing Assessment (Reason)	Nursing Diagnosis (Problem)	Expected Outcome (Objective)	Nursing Interventions	Rationale	Evaluation
Subjective data: .... Objective data:					

Contd...

Contd...

Nursing Assessment (Reason)	Nursing Diagnosis (Problem)	Expected Outcome (Objective)	Nursing Interventions	Rationale	Evaluation
Subjective data: .... Objective data:					

NURSING CARE PLAN NO. 4

Note 1: Students are advised to write at least 10 points on nursing care plan for selected case study and case presentation.

Note 2: Students are advised to write nursing care plan for the patient' problem or nursing diagnosis on priority basis with at least 5–6 identified actual or potential problems, and can also state accordingly short- or long-term goals and intervention accordingly.

Name of the Patient: ....

Age: ....

Sex: ....

Diagnosis: ....

Date of Care Started:

Nursing Assessment (Reason)	Nursing Diagnosis (Problem)	Expected Outcome (Objective)	Nursing Interventions	Rationale	Evaluation
Subjective data: .... Objective data:					

Contd...

Contd...

Nursing Assessment (Reason)	Nursing Diagnosis (Problem)	Expected Outcome (Objective)	Nursing Interventions	Rationale	Evaluation
Subjective data: .... Objective data:					

NURSING CARE PLAN NO. 5

Note 1: Students are advised to write at least 10 points on nursing care plan for selected case study and case presentation.

Note 2: Students are advised to write nursing care plan for the patient' problem or nursing diagnosis on priority basis with at least 5–6 identified actual or potential problems, and can also state accordingly short- or long-term goals and intervention accordingly.

Name of the Patient: ....

Age: ....

Sex: ....

Diagnosis: ....

Date of Care Started:

Nursing Assessment (Reason)	Nursing Diagnosis (Problem)	Expected Outcome (Objective)	Nursing Interventions	Rationale	Evaluation
Subjective data: .... Objective data:					

Contd...

Contd...

Nursing Assessment (Reason)	Nursing Diagnosis (Problem)	Expected Outcome (Objective)	Nursing Interventions	Rationale	Evaluation
Subjective data: .... Objective data:					

NURSING CARE PLAN NO. 6

Note 1: Students are advised to write at least 10 points on nursing care plan for selected case study and case presentation.

Note 2: Students are advised to write nursing care plan for the patient' problem or nursing diagnosis on priority basis with at least 5–6 identified actual or potential problems, and can also state accordingly short- or long-term goals and intervention accordingly.

Name of the Patient: ....

Age: ....

Sex: ....

Diagnosis: ....

Date of Care Started:

Nursing Assessment (Reason)	Nursing Diagnosis (Problem)	Expected Outcome (Objective)	Nursing Interventions	Rationale	Evaluation
Subjective data: .... Objective data:					

Contd...

Contd...

Nursing Assessment (Reason)	Nursing Diagnosis (Problem)	Expected Outcome (Objective)	Nursing Interventions	Rationale	Evaluation
Subjective data: .... Objective data:					

NURSING CARE PLAN NO. 7

Note 1: Students are advised to write at least 10 points on nursing care plan for selected case study and case presentation.

Note 2: Students are advised to write nursing care plan for the patient' problem or nursing diagnosis on priority basis with at least 5–6 identified actual or potential problems, and can also state accordingly short- or long-term goals and intervention accordingly.

Name of the Patient: ....

Age: ....

Sex: ....

Diagnosis: ....

Date of Care Started:

Nursing Assessment (Reason)	Nursing Diagnosis (Problem)	Expected Outcome (Objective)	Nursing Interventions	Rationale	Evaluation
Subjective data: .... Objective data:					

Contd...

Contd...

Nursing Assessment (Reason)	Nursing Diagnosis (Problem)	Expected Outcome (Objective)	Nursing Interventions	Rationale	Evaluation
Subjective data: .... Objective data:					

NURSING CARE PLAN NO. 8

Note 1: Students are advised to write at least 10 points on nursing care plan for selected case study and case presentation.

Note 2: Students are advised to write nursing care plan for the patient' problem or nursing diagnosis on priority basis with at least 5–6 identified actual or potential problems, and can also state accordingly short- or long-term goals and intervention accordingly.

Name of the Patient: ....

Age: ....

Sex: ....

Diagnosis: ....

Date of Care Started:

Nursing Assessment (Reason)	Nursing Diagnosis (Problem)	Expected Outcome (Objective)	Nursing Interventions	Rationale	Evaluation
Subjective data: .... Objective data:					

Contd...

Contd...

Nursing Assessment (Reason)	Nursing Diagnosis (Problem)	Expected Outcome (Objective)	Nursing Interventions	Rationale	Evaluation
Subjective data: .... Objective data:					

NURSING CARE PLAN NO. 9

Note 1: Students are advised to write at least 10 points on nursing care plan for selected case study and case presentation.

Note 2: Students are advised to write nursing care plan for the patient' problem or nursing diagnosis on priority basis with at least 5–6 identified actual or potential problems, and can also state accordingly short- or long-term goals and intervention accordingly.

Name of the Patient: ....

Age: ....

Sex: ....

Diagnosis: ....

Date of Care Started:

Nursing Assessment (Reason)	Nursing Diagnosis (Problem)	Expected Outcome (Objective)	Nursing Interventions	Rationale	Evaluation
Subjective data: .... Objective data:					

Contd...

Contd...

Nursing Assessment (Reason)	Nursing Diagnosis (Problem)	Expected Outcome (Objective)	Nursing Interventions	Rationale	Evaluation
Subjective data: .... Objective data:					

NURSING CARE PLAN NO. 10

Note 1: Students are advised to write at least 10 points on nursing care plan for selected case study and case presentation.

Note 2: Students are advised to write nursing care plan for the patient' problem or nursing diagnosis on priority basis with at least 5–6 identified actual or potential problems, and can also state accordingly short- or long-term goals and intervention accordingly.

Name of the Patient: ....

Age: ....

Sex: ....

Diagnosis: ....

Date of Care Started:

Nursing Assessment (Reason)	Nursing Diagnosis (Problem)	Expected Outcome (Objective)	Nursing Interventions	Rationale	Evaluation
Subjective data: .... Objective data:					

Contd...

Contd...

Nursing Assessment (Reason)	Nursing Diagnosis (Problem)	Expected Outcome (Objective)	Nursing Interventions	Rationale	Evaluation
Subjective data: .... Objective data:					

NURSING CARE PLAN NO. 11

Note 1: Students are advised to write at least 10 points on nursing care plan for selected case study and case presentation.

Note 2: Students are advised to write nursing care plan for the patient' problem or nursing diagnosis on priority basis with at least 5–6 identified actual or potential problems, and can also state accordingly short- or long-term goals and intervention accordingly.

Name of the Patient: ....

Age: ....

Sex: ....

Diagnosis: ....

Date of Care Started:

Nursing Assessment (Reason)	Nursing Diagnosis (Problem)	Expected Outcome (Objective)	Nursing Interventions	Rationale	Evaluation
Subjective data: .... Objective data:					

Contd...

Contd...

Nursing Assessment (Reason)	Nursing Diagnosis (Problem)	Expected Outcome (Objective)	Nursing Interventions	Rationale	Evaluation
Subjective data: .... Objective data:					

NURSING CARE PLAN NO. 12

Note 1: Students are advised to write at least 10 points on nursing care plan for selected case study and case presentation.

Note 2: Students are advised to write nursing care plan for the patient' problem or nursing diagnosis on priority basis with at least 5–6 identified actual or potential problems, and can also state accordingly short- or long-term goals and intervention accordingly.

Name of the Patient: ....

Age: ....

Sex: ....

Diagnosis: ....

Date of Care Started:

Nursing Assessment (Reason)	Nursing Diagnosis (Problem)	Expected Outcome (Objective)	Nursing Interventions	Rationale	Evaluation
Subjective data: .... Objective data:					

Contd...

Contd...

Nursing Assessment (Reason)	**Nursing Diagnosis (Problem)**	**Expected Outcome (Objective)**	**Nursing Interventions**	**Rationale**	**Evaluation**
Subjective data: .... Objective data:					

NURSING CARE PLAN NO. 13

Note 1: Students are advised to write at least 10 points on nursing care plan for selected case study and case presentation.

Note 2: Students are advised to write nursing care plan for the patient' problem or nursing diagnosis on priority basis with at least 5–6 identified actual or potential problems, and can also state accordingly short- or long-term goals and intervention accordingly.

Name of the Patient: ....

Age: ....

Sex: ....

Diagnosis: ....

Date of Care Started:

Nursing Assessment (Reason)	Nursing Diagnosis (Problem)	Expected Outcome (Objective)	Nursing Interventions	Rationale	Evaluation
Subjective data: .... Objective data:					

Contd...

Contd...

Nursing Assessment (Reason)	Nursing Diagnosis (Problem)	Expected Outcome (Objective)	Nursing Interventions	Rationale	Evaluation
Subjective data: .... Objective data:					

NURSING CARE PLAN NO. 14

Note 1: Students are advised to write at least 10 points on nursing care plan for selected case study and case presentation.

Note 2: Students are advised to write nursing care plan for the patient' problem or nursing diagnosis on priority basis with at least 5–6 identified actual or potential problems, and can also state accordingly short- or long-term goals and intervention accordingly.

Name of the Patient: ....

Age: ....

Sex: ....

Diagnosis: ....

Date of Care Started:

Nursing Assessment (Reason)	Nursing Diagnosis (Problem)	Expected Outcome (Objective)	Nursing Interventions	Rationale	Evaluation
Subjective data: .... Objective data:					

Contd...

Contd...

Nursing Assessment (Reason)	Nursing Diagnosis (Problem)	Expected Outcome (Objective)	Nursing Interventions	Rationale	Evaluation
Subjective data: .... Objective data:					

NURSING CARE PLAN NO. 15

Note 1: Students are advised to write at least 10 points on nursing care plan for selected case study and case presentation.

Note 2: Students are advised to write nursing care plan for the patient' problem or nursing diagnosis on priority basis with at least 5–6 identified actual or potential problems, and can also state accordingly short- or long-term goals and intervention accordingly.

Name of the Patient: ....

Age: ....

Sex: ....

Diagnosis: ....

Date of Care Started:

Nursing Assessment (Reason)	Nursing Diagnosis (Problem)	Expected Outcome (Objective)	Nursing Interventions	Rationale	Evaluation
Subjective data: .... Objective data:					

Contd...

Contd...

Nursing Assessment (Reason)	Nursing Diagnosis (Problem)	Expected Outcome (Objective)	Nursing Interventions	Rationale	Evaluation
Subjective data: .... Objective data:					

SECTION V

DRUG BOOK

1. Study of Specific Drug

Trade Name: ....

Generic Name: ....

Drug Group: ....

Action of the Drug: ....

....

....

Indications of the Drug: ....

Dosage: ....

Route of Administration: ....

Side Effects:

....

....

....

Contraindications:

....

....

....

Nurses Responsibilities:

....

....

....

....

....

References: Example, Nursing Drug Book. New Delhi: Jaypee Brothers Medical Publisher (P) Ltd; 2014.

DRUG BOOK

2. Study of Specific Drug

Trade Name: ....

Generic Name: ....

Drug Group: ....

Action of the Drug: ....

....

....

Indications of the Drug: ....

Dosage: ....

Route of Administration: ....

Side Effects:

....

....

....

Contraindications:

....

....

....

Nurses Responsibilities:

....

....

....

....

....

References: Example, Nursing Drug Book. New Delhi: Jaypee Brothers Medical Publisher (P) Ltd; 2014.

DRUG BOOK

3. Study of Specific Drug

Trade Name: ....

Generic Name: ....

Drug Group: ....

Action of the Drug: ....

....

....

Indications of the Drug: ....

Dosage: ....

Route of Administration: ....

Side Effects:

....

....

....

Contraindications:

....

....

....

Nurses Responsibilities:

....

....

....

....

....

References: Example, Nursing Drug Book. New Delhi: Jaypee Brothers Medical Publisher (P) Ltd; 2014.

DRUG BOOK

4. Study of Specific Drug

Trade Name: ....

Generic Name: ....

Drug Group: ....

Action of the Drug: ....

....

....

Indications of the Drug: ....

Dosage: ....

Route of Administration: ....

Side Effects:

....

....

....

Contraindications:

....

....

....

Nurses Responsibilities:

....

....

....

....

....

References: Example, Nursing Drug Book. New Delhi: Jaypee Brothers Medical Publisher (P) Ltd; 2014.

DRUG BOOK

5. Study of Specific Drug

Trade Name: ....

Generic Name: ....

Drug Group: ....

Action of the Drug: ....

....

....

Indications of the Drug: ....

Dosage: ....

Route of Administration: ....

Side Effects:

....

....

....

Contraindications:

....

....

....

Nurses Responsibilities:

....

....

....

....

....

References: Example, Nursing Drug Book. New Delhi: Jaypee Brothers Medical Publisher (P) Ltd; 2014.

DRUG BOOK

6. Study of Specific Drug

Trade Name: ....

Generic Name: ....

Drug Group: ....

Action of the Drug: ....

....

....

Indications of the Drug: ....

Dosage: ....

Route of Administration: ....

Side Effects:

....

....

....

Contraindications:

....

....

....

Nurses Responsibilities:

....

....

....

....

....

References: Example, Nursing Drug Book. New Delhi: Jaypee Brothers Medical Publisher (P) Ltd; 2014.

DRUG BOOK

7. Study of Specific Drug

Trade Name: ....

Generic Name: ....

Drug Group: ....

Action of the Drug: ....

....

....

Indications of the Drug: ....

Dosage: ....

Route of Administration: ....

Side Effects:

....

....

....

Contraindications:

....

....

....

Nurses Responsibilities:

....

....

....

....

....

References: Example, Nursing Drug Book. New Delhi: Jaypee Brothers Medical Publisher (P) Ltd; 2014.

DRUG BOOK

8. Study of Specific Drug

Trade Name: ....

Generic Name: ....

Drug Group: ....

Action of the Drug: ....

....

....

Indications of the Drug: ....

Dosage: ....

Route of Administration: ....

Side Effects:

....

....

....

Contraindications:

....

....

....

Nurses Responsibilities:

....

....

....

....

....

References: Example, Nursing Drug Book. New Delhi: Jaypee Brothers Medical Publisher (P) Ltd; 2014.

DRUG BOOK

9. Study of Specific Drug

Trade Name: ....

Generic Name: ....

Drug Group: ....

Action of the Drug: ....

....

....

Indications of the Drug: ....

Dosage: ....

Route of Administration: ....

Side Effects:

....

....

....

Contraindications:

....

....

....

Nurses Responsibilities:

....

....

....

....

....

References: Example, Nursing Drug Book. New Delhi: Jaypee Brothers Medical Publisher (P) Ltd; 2014.

DRUG BOOK

10. Study of Specific Drug

Trade Name: ....

Generic Name: ....

Drug Group: ....

Action of the Drug: ....

....

....

Indications of the Drug: ....

Dosage: ....

Route of Administration: ....

Side Effects:

....

....

....

Contraindications:

....

....

....

Nurses Responsibilities:

....

....

....

....

....

References: Example, Nursing Drug Book. New Delhi: Jaypee Brothers Medical Publisher (P) Ltd; 2014.

LIST OF DRUGS USED DURING CLINICAL EXPERIENCE

Note: Students are instructed to write drugs used for different patients during the clinical experience as the format given below.

SI No	Date	Patient's Name	Medication	Indication	Dosage/Route/ Frequency	Side Effects	Contraind- ications	Nurses Responsibilities

SECTION VI

HEALTH TALK-1

Name of Student Teacher : Year:

Name of Supervisor :

Subject :

Topic :

Group and Size :

Date and Time :

Venue :

Method of Teaching : Audiovisual (AV) Aids:

Method of Evaluation :

Previous Knowledge of the Group:

General Objectives:

Specific Objectives:

Bibliography

1.
2.
3.

FORMAT OF HEALTH TALK

Time	Specific Objective	Content	Teacher's Activity	Learner's Activity	Audiovisual (AV)Aids	Evaluation

Summary and Conclusion:

HEALTH TALK-2

Name of Student Teacher : Year:

Name of Supervisor :

Subject :

Topic :

Group and Size :

Date and Time :

Venue :

Method of Teaching : Audiovisual (AV) Aids:

Method of Evaluation :

Previous Knowledge of the Group:

General Objectives:

Specific Objectives:

Bibliography

1.

2.

3.

FORMAT OF HEALTH TALK

Time	Specific Objective	Content	Teacher's Activity	Learner's Activity	Audiovisual (AV)Aids	Evaluation

Summary and Conclusion:

HEALTH TALK-3

Name of Student Teacher : Year:

Name of Supervisor :

Subject :

Topic :

Group and Size :

Date and Time :

Venue :

Method of Teaching : Audiovisual (AV) Aids:

Method of Evaluation :

Previous Knowledge of the Group:

General Objectives:

Specific Objectives:

Bibliography

1.

2.

3.

FORMAT OF HEALTH TALK

Time	Specific Objective	Content	Teacher's Activity	Learner's Activity	Audiovisual (AV)Aids	Evaluation

Summary and Conclusion:

HEALTH TALK-4

Name of Student Teacher : Year:

Name of Supervisor :

Subject :

Topic :

Group and Size :

Date and Time :

Venue :

Method of Teaching : Audiovisual (AV) Aids:

Method of Evaluation :

Previous Knowledge of the Group:

General Objectives:

Specific Objectives:

Bibliography

1.
2.
3.

FORMAT OF HEALTH TALK

Time	Specific Objective	Content	Teacher's Activity	Learner's Activity	Audiovisual (AV)Aids	Evaluation

Summary and Conclusion:

HEALTH TALK-5

Name of Student Teacher : Year:

Name of Supervisor :

Subject :

Topic :

Group and Size :

Date and Time :

Venue :

Method of Teaching : Audiovisual (AV) Aids:

Method of Evaluation :

Previous Knowledge of the Group:

General Objectives:

Specific Objectives:

Bibliography

1.
2.
3.

FORMAT OF HEALTH TALK

Time	Specific Objective	Content	Teacher's Activity	Learner's Activity	Audiovisual (AV)Aids	Evaluation

Summary and Conclusion:

SECTION VII

BEDSIDE DEMONSTRATION-1

Identification Data of Patient

(Introduce the patient with name, age, address, religion, his/her marital status, socioeconomic status, he/she is admitted to hospital, onset of illness, presented signs and symptoms, history of previous illness, treatment, etc.)

Definition of disease:

Nursing assessment: Mention key points of subjective data and objective data, and nursing diagnosis and problem.

Nursing diagnosis: List of problem on the basis of priority of patient:

1.
2.
3.
4.
5.
6.
7.
8.
9.
10.

Planning: State the objectives of care:

1.
2.
3.
4.
5.
6.

Intervention: State the nursing intervention performed to be performed

1.
2.
3.
4.
5.
6.

Nursing procedure: Related to patient condition

- Name of the procedure:

- Definition of the procedure:

- Purposes of the procedure:

- Articles required:

1.
2.
3.
4.
5.
6.
7.
8.
9.

- Preparation of the patients:

1.
2.
3.
4.
5.
6.
7.
8.
9.
10.

- Key steps of the procedure with rationale: ....

- Care of the patient after the procedure: ....

- Care of the articles/area: ....

- Comments: ....

Health teaching: ....

BEDSIDE DEMONSTRATION-2

Identification Data of Patient

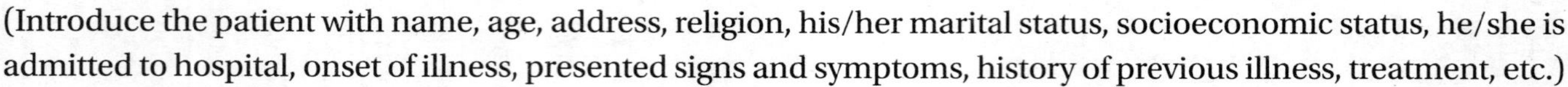

(Introduce the patient with name, age, address, religion, his/her marital status, socioeconomic status, he/she is admitted to hospital, onset of illness, presented signs and symptoms, history of previous illness, treatment, etc.)

Definition of disease:

Nursing assessment: Mention key points of subjective data and objective data, and nursing diagnosis and problem.

Nursing diagnosis: List of problem on the basis of priority of patient:

1.
2.
3.
4.
5.
6.
7.
8.
9.
10.

Planning: State the objectives of care:

1.
2.
3.
4.
5.
6.

Intervention: State the nursing intervention performed to be performed

1.
2.
3.
4.
5.
6.

Nursing procedure: Related to patient condition

- Name of the procedure:

- Definition of the procedure:

- Purposes of the procedure:

- Articles required:

1.
2.
3.
4.
5.
6.
7.
8.
9.

- Preparation of the patients:

1.
2.
3.
4.
5.
6.
7.
8.
9.
10.

- Key steps of the procedure with rationale: ....

- Care of the patient after the procedure: ....

- Care of the articles/area: ....

- Comments: ....

Health teaching: ....

BEDSIDE DEMONSTRATION-3

Identification Data of Patient

(Introduce the patient with name, age, address, religion, his/her marital status, socioeconomic status, he/she is admitted to hospital, onset of illness, presented signs and symptoms, history of previous illness, treatment, etc.)

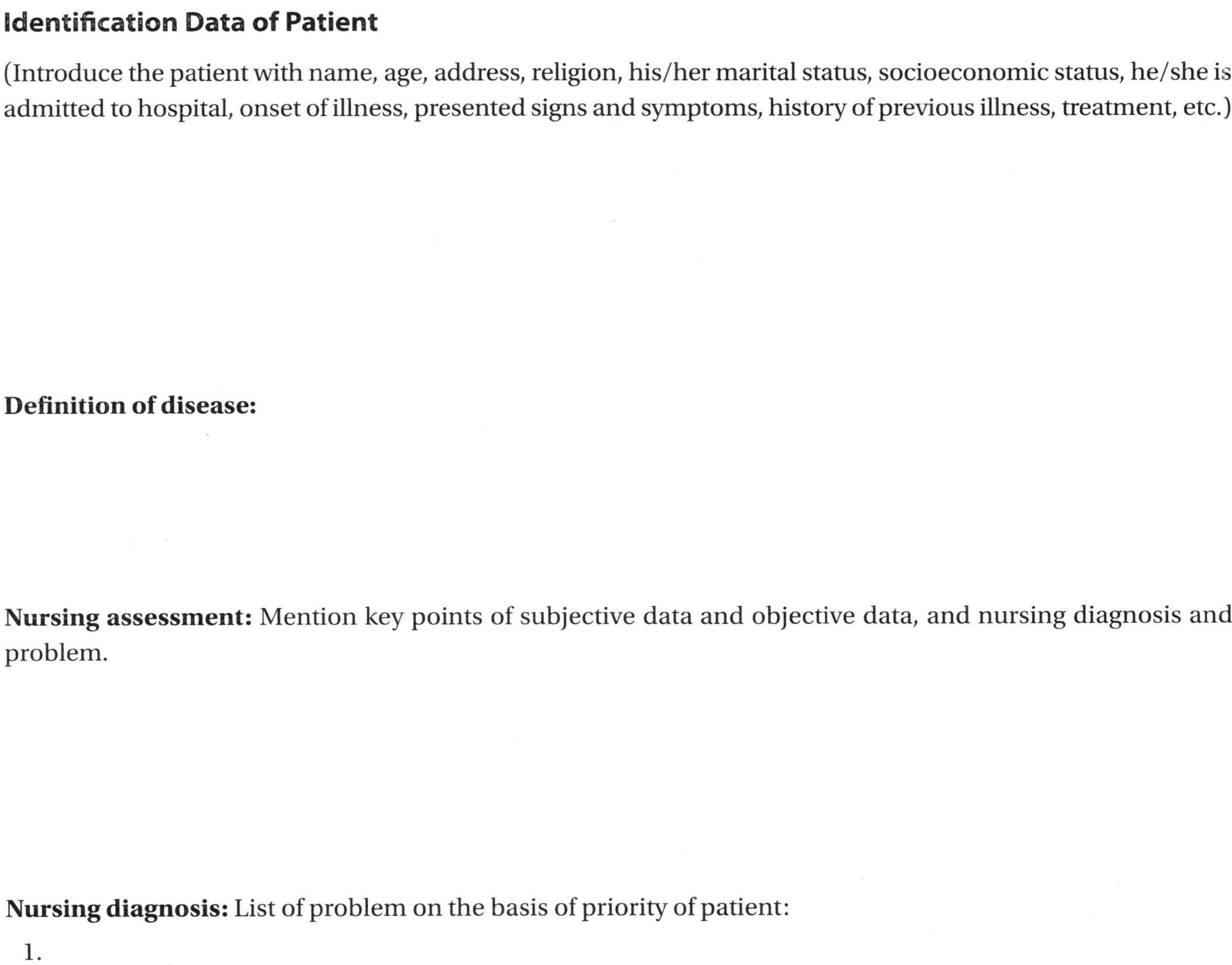

Definition of disease:

Nursing assessment: Mention key points of subjective data and objective data, and nursing diagnosis and problem.

Nursing diagnosis: List of problem on the basis of priority of patient:

1.
2.
3.
4.
5.
6.
7.
8.
9.
10.

Planning: State the objectives of care:

1.
2.
3.
4.
5.
6.

Intervention: State the nursing intervention performed to be performed

1.
2.
3.
4.
5.
6.

Nursing procedure: Related to patient condition

- Name of the procedure:

- Definition of the procedure:

- Purposes of the procedure:

- Articles required:

1.
2.
3.
4.
5.
6.
7.
8.
9.

- Preparation of the patients:

1.
2.
3.
4.
5.
6.
7.
8.
9.
10.

- Key steps of the procedure with rationale: ....

- Care of the patient after the procedure: ....

- Care of the articles/area: ....

- Comments: ....

Health teaching: ....

BEDSIDE DEMONSTRATION-4

Identification Data of Patient

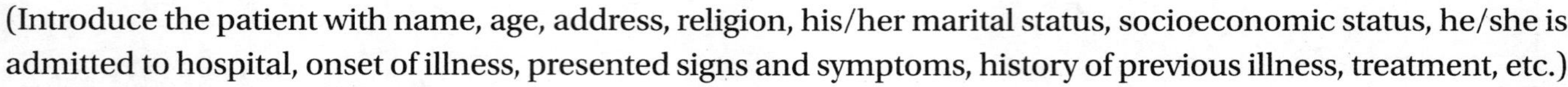

(Introduce the patient with name, age, address, religion, his/her marital status, socioeconomic status, he/she is admitted to hospital, onset of illness, presented signs and symptoms, history of previous illness, treatment, etc.)

Definition of disease:

Nursing assessment: Mention key points of subjective data and objective data, and nursing diagnosis and problem.

Nursing diagnosis: List of problem on the basis of priority of patient:

1.
2.
3.
4.
5.
6.
7.
8.
9.
10.

Planning: State the objectives of care:

1.
2.
3.
4.
5.
6.

Intervention: State the nursing intervention performed to be performed

1.
2.
3.
4.
5.
6.

Nursing procedure: Related to patient condition

- Name of the procedure:

- Definition of the procedure:

- Purposes of the procedure:

- Articles required:

1.
2.
3.
4.
5.
6.
7.
8.
9.

- Preparation of the patients:

1.
2.
3.
4.
5.
6.
7.
8.
9.
10.

- Key steps of the procedure with rationale: ....

- Care of the patient after the procedure: ....

- Care of the articles/area: ....

- Comments: ....

Health teaching: ....

BEDSIDE DEMONSTRATION-5

Identification Data of Patient

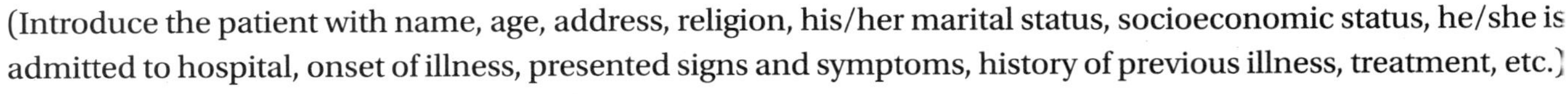

(Introduce the patient with name, age, address, religion, his/her marital status, socioeconomic status, he/she is admitted to hospital, onset of illness, presented signs and symptoms, history of previous illness, treatment, etc.)

Definition of disease:

Nursing assessment: Mention key points of subjective data and objective data, and nursing diagnosis and problem.

Nursing diagnosis: List of problem on the basis of priority of patient:

1.
2.
3.
4.
5.
6.
7.
8.
9.
10.

Planning: State the objectives of care:

1.
2.
3.
4.
5.
6.

Intervention: State the nursing intervention performed to be performed

1.
2.
3.
4.
5.
6.

Nursing procedure: Related to patient condition

- Name of the procedure:
- Definition of the procedure:
- Purposes of the procedure:
- Articles required:

1.
2.
3.
4.
5.
6.
7.
8.
9.

- Preparation of the patients:

1.
2.
3.
4.
5.
6.
7.
8.
9.
10.

- Key steps of the procedure with rationale: ....

- Care of the patient after the procedure: ....

- Care of the articles/area: ....

- Comments: ....

Health teaching: ....

SECTION VIII

INTENSIVE CARE UNIT

Report of Experience in Intensive Care Unit

General Objectives:

Principles of Intensive Care Unit (ICU):

Physical Layout/Set (Draw a Diagram of ICU):

List of Equipment Used in ICU:

Name of the Equipment	Purpose

List of Procedures Performed in ICU:

Name of the Procedures	Purposes	Indications	Nurses Responsibility Assisted/ Performed

List of Drugs used in ICU:

Name of the Drugs	Route/Dosage	Action	Side Effects	Nurses Responsibility

Nurses Responsibility in ICU:

1.
2.
3.
4.
5.
6.

Summary of Student Experience in ICU:

SECTION IX

OPERATION THEATER

Report of Experience in Operation Theater

General Objectives:

Physical Layout Setup (Draw a Diagram of Physical Layout):

Method of Sterilization of Equipment/Linen in Operation Theater (OT):

Sterilization:

- Blunt instruments:
- Sharp instruments:
- Linen:
- Chemicals used:

Autoclaving Method:

Linen:

Instruments:

Fumigation (Chemical used):

Medical Asepsis:

Universal precautions followed:

Surgical Asepsis: Scrubbing

Universal precautions followed:

Setting up of Trolley for Operation (General or Specific)

List the articles, instrument and their purposes:

1.
2.
3.
4.
5.
6.
7.
8.
9.
10.

List the Surgeries Witnessed or Assisted

Name of the Patients	Age	Sex	Diagnoses	Anesthesia Type used Local Anesthesia (LA)/General Anesthesia (GA)/Epidural Analgesia

List the Common Drugs used in Operation Theater with the Purposes

Name of the Drugs	Indication	Action	Dosage	Side Effects

List the Nurses Responsibility in Operation Theater

1.
2.
3.
4.
5.
6.
7.
8.
9.
10.

Preoperative Care (What has been Performed/Done):

Postoperative Care (What has been Performed/Done):

Conclusion:

References:

1.
2.
3.
4.
5.

SECTION X

CRITERIA FOR EVALUATION OF CLINICAL EXPERIENCE

Name of the Student:

Name of the Hospital:

Name of the Ward/Unit:

Name of the Supervisor/HOD:

I. CASE STUDY

Max. Marks: 25

Sl No	Content	Marks Allotted	Marks Obtained	Remarks
1.	History taking	02		
2.	Physical examination	02		
3.	Medication	02		
4.	Disease condition	05		
5.	Nursing care plan	08		
6.	Health education	02		
7.	Summary and conclusion	02		
Total		**25**		

II. CASE PRESENTATION

Max. Marks: 25

Sl No	Content	Marks Allotted	Marks Obtained	Remarks
1.	Content organization	08		
2.	Preparing environment	05		
3.	AV aids	05		
4.	Summary	01		
5.	Conclusion	01		
6.	Bibliography	01		
Total		**25**		

III. NURSING CARE PLAN

Max. Marks: 25

Sl No	Content	Marks Allotted	Marks Obtained	Remarks
1.	History taking	04		
2.	Priority of needs/problems	04		
3.	Nursing process	10		
4.	Diet planning	03		
5.	Health teaching	02		
6.	Bibliography	02		
Total		**25**		

IV. BEDSIDE DEMONSTRATION

Max. Marks: 25

Sl No	Content	Marks Allotted	Marks Obtained	Remarks
1.	Assessment of Patient	02		
2.	Principle used in procedures	02		
3.	Preparation of patient environment, equipment	04		
4.	Steps of procedure	07		
5.	Care of patient, equipment and environment of patient	04		
6.	Bibliography	01		
	Total	**25**		

V. OT REPORT

Max. Marks: 25

Sl No	Content	Marks Allotted	Marks Obtained	Remarks
1.	Physical setting	02		
2.	Daily routine	02		
3.	Procedures	02		
4.	Emergency medication trolley	03		
5.	Instrument using	03		
6.	Operating machine	03		
7.	Knowledge and application	03		
8.	Nurses responsibility	05		
9.	Bibliography	02		
	Total	**25**		

VI. ICU REPORT

Max. Marks: 50

Sl No	Content	Marks Allotted	Marks Obtained	Remarks
1.	Physical set-up	05		
2.	Medication	05		
3.	Instruments application	05		
4.	General trolley setup	05		
5.	Anesthesia trolley	05		
6.	Witness and assisting case	10		
7.	Pre- and post-operative care	10		
8.	Nurses responsibility	05		
	Total	**50**		

VII. HEALTH TALK

Max. Marks: 25

Sl No	Content	Marks Allotted	Marks Obtained	Remarks
1.	Objective, structure	03		
2.	Content organization	05		
3.	Principles of teaching journals	05		
4.	Presentation of content	05		
5.	Groups response	03		
6.	AV aids	02		
7.	Bibliography	02		
Total		**25**		

EVALUATION OF TOTAL CLINICAL EXPERIENCE

Sl No	Content	Marks Allotted	Marks Obtained	Remarks
1.	Case study	25		
2.	Case presentation	25		
3.	Nursing care plan	25		
4.	Bedside demonstration	25		
5.	OT report	25		
6.	ICU report	50		
7.	Health talk	25		
Grand Total		**200**		

Signature of Student

Date:

Signature of Supervisor

Date: